DR. SEBI DIET

The Ultimate Guide On How To Detox The Liver, Cleanse Your Body, Reverse Disease Through Alkaline Diet Method

By

Anna Watson

© **Copyright 2019 by Anna Watson**

All rights reserved.

This document is geared towards providing exact and reliable information with regards to the topic and issue covered. The publication is sold with the idea that the publisher is not required to render accounting, officially permitted, or otherwise, qualified services. If advice is necessary, legal or professional, a practiced individual in the profession should be ordered.

From a Declaration of Principles which was accepted and approved equally by a Committee of the American Bar Association and a Committee of Publishers and Associations.

In no way is it legal to reproduce, duplicate, or transmit any part of this document in either electronic means or in printed format. Recording of this publication is strictly prohibited and any storage of this document is not allowed unless with written permission from the publisher. All rights reserved.

The information provided herein is stated to be truthful and consistent, in that any liability, in terms of inattention or otherwise, by any usage or abuse of any policies, processes, or directions contained within is the solitary and utter responsibility of the recipient reader. Under no circumstances will any legal responsibility or blame be held against the publisher for any reparation, damages, or monetary loss due to the information herein, either directly or indirectly.

Respective authors own all copyrights not held by the publisher.

The information herein is offered for informational purposes solely, and is universal as so. The presentation of the information is without contract or any type of guarantee assurance.

The trademarks that are used are without any consent, and the publication of the trademark is without permission or backing by the trademark owner. All trademarks and brands within this book are for clarifying purposes only and are the owned by the owners themselves, not affiliated with this document.

DISCLAIMER

All erudition contained in this book is given for informational and educational purposes only. The author is not in any way accountable for any results or outcomes that emanate from using this material. Constructive attempts have been made to provide information that is both accurate and effective, but the author is not bound for the accuracy or use/misuse of this information.

TABLE OF CONTENTS

Introduction 1
Chapter One: What Is The Dr. Sebi Alkaline Diet? 3
Chapter Two: Benefits Of The Alkaline Diet 53
Chapter Three: The Alkaline Diet Method And Weight Loss 99
Chapter Four: Detoxing The Liver 139

INTRODUCTION

The Dr. Sebi alkaline diet is otherwise called the ph. wonder, ph. balance diet, or the acid-alkaline food in addition to other things. It was dependent on the theory that everything that you eat can either make your body develop acid or to turn out to be progressively alkaline. For somebody beginning this diet, it very well may be overpowering, attempting to make sense of what is excellent (alkaline) and what is terrible (acidic). There are many basic diet rules.

The essential thought is certain substances are more terrible for the body than others. The Dr. Sebi basic diet rules is that you should endeavor to eat 75-80% alkaline. You are implying that 75-80% of your diet is from the basic nourishment outline. Certain nourishments are viewed as more acid framing than others. To give you a thought here is a rundown of nourishments that are considered as exceptionally acid framing as indicated by the alkaline diet rules: sugars (equivalent, sweet and low, and aspartame to give some examples) lager, table salt, jam, frozen yogurt, hamburger, lobster, singed nourishment, prepared cheddar, and soda pops. Here is a fun actuality cola has a ph. of 2.5. This is profoundly acidic. To kill on the jar of cola, you would need to drink 32 glasses of water.

On the opposite side of the range, there is sure nourishment that is considered to be profoundly alkaline and, when ingested, helps increment the alkalinity of the body. As per the Dr. Sebi diet rules, this nourishment is as per the following: ocean salt, lotus rood, watermelon, tangerines, sweet potato, lime, pineapple, kelp, pumpkin seeds, and lentils. The basic diet rules state that drugs are incredibly acid shaping too.

Consider each one of those individuals who take some drugs to facilitate their acid reflux. Much to their dismay, their impermanent arrangement is causing more severe issues for them over the long haul. There are numerous other Dr. Sebi alkaline diet nourishments; this was only a model. The more you eat, the better you will feel. Commonly individuals experience a time of detoxification when they change to the Dr. Sebi alkaline diet. The salty diet rules recommend that you overcame a time of a long time in detox to free your assortment of poisons and permit you to conform to this better approach for eating.

CHAPTER ONE
WHAT IS THE DR. SEBI ALKALINE DIET?

The Dr. Sebi diet

The Dr. Sebi diet, likewise called the Dr. Sebi alkaline diet, is a plant-based diet created by the late Dr. Sebi. It's professed to revive your cells by dispensing with harmful waste through alkalizing your blood. The menu depends on eating a short rundown of endorsed nourishments alongside numerous enhancements. This article audits the advantages and drawbacks of the Dr. Sebi diet and whether logical proof backs up its health claims.

What is Dr. Sebi's diet?

This diet depends on the African Bio-Mineral Balance theory and was created by oneself instructed botanist Alfredo Darrington Bowman — otherwise called Dr. Sebi. Regardless of his name, Dr. Sebi was not a medicinal specialist and didn't hold a Ph.D. He planned this diet for any individual who wishes to usually fix or counteract disease and improve their general health without depending on the conventional Western drug. As indicated by Dr. Sebi, the condition is an aftereffect of bodily fluid develop in a region of your body. For instance, the development of bodily fluid in the lungs is pneumonia, while abundance bodily fluid in the pancreas is diabetes. He contends that diseases can't exist in an alkaline domain and start to happen when your body turns out to be excessively acidic. By carefully following his diet and utilizing his restrictive exorbitant enhancements, he vows to re-establish your body's natural alkaline state and detoxify your diseased body. Initially, Dr. Sebi guaranteed that this diet could fix conditions like AIDS, sickle cell paleness, leukemia, and lupus. In any case, after a 1993 claim, he was requested to stop making such claims. The diet comprises of a particular rundown of affirmed vegetables, natural products, grains, nuts, seeds, oils, and herbs. As creature items are not allowed, the Dr. Sebi diet is viewed as a veggie lover diet. Sebi asserted that for your body to recuperate itself, you should pursue the menu reliably for a mind-blowing remainder. At last, while numerous individuals demand that the program has mended them, no logical investigations bolster these cases. The Dr. Sebi diet underscores expending nourishments and enhancements that, as far as anyone knows, decline disease-causing bodily fluid by accomplishing an alkaline state in your body.

Step by step instructions to pursue the Dr. Sebi diet

As indicated by Dr. Sebi's wholesome guide, you should keep these essential guidelines:

Rule 1. You should eat nourishments recorded in the healthful guide.

Rule 2. Drink 1 gallon (3.8 liters) of water each day.

Rule 3. Take Dr. Sebi's enhancements an hour before prescriptions.

Rule 4. No creature items are allowed.

Rule 5. No liquor is permitted.

Rule 6. Stay away from wheat items and devour the "regular developing grains" recorded in the guide.

Rule 7. Abstain from utilizing a microwave to counteract murdering your nourishment.

Rule 8. Stay away from canned or seedless organic products.

There are no particular supplement rules. In any case, this diet is low in protein, as it precludes beans, lentils, and creature and soy items. Protein is a significant supplement required for solid muscles, skin, and joints. Furthermore, you're required to buy Dr. Sebi's cell nourishment items, which are supplements that guarantee to cleanse your body and support your cells. It's prescribed to purchase the "comprehensive" bundle, which contains 20 distinct items that are professed to cleanse and reestablish your whole body at the quickest rate conceivable. Other than this, no particular enhancement suggestions are given. Instead, you're relied upon to arrange any enhancement that matches your health concerns. For instance, the "Bio Ferro" cases guarantee to treat liver issues, cleanse your blood, support insusceptibility, advance weight loss, help stomach related problems, and increment generally prosperity.

Moreover, the enhancements don't contain a total rundown of supplements or their amounts, making it hard to tell whether they will meet your everyday needs. The Dr. Sebi diet has eight primary standards that must be pursued. They, for the most part, center on maintaining a strategic distance from creature items, ultra-handled nourishment, and taking his exclusive enhancements. This diet has a severe rundown of permitted nourishments. Nourishments that are excluded from this rundown ought to be maintained a strategic distance from.

Nourishments to dodge

Any nourishments that are excluded from the Dr. Sebi sustenance direct are not allowed, for example,

- Canned natural product or vegetables
- Seedless natural product
- Eggs
- Dairy

- Fish
- Red meat
- Poultry
- Soy items
- processed nourishment, including take-out or café nourishment
- fortified nourishments
- Wheat
- Sugar (other than date sugar and agave syrup)
- Alcohol
- Yeast or nourishments ascended with yeast.
- Foods made with heating powder.

Besides, many vegetables, natural products, grains, nuts, and seeds are prohibited on a diet.

Just nourishments recorded in the guide might be eaten. As far as possible, any nourishment that is handled, creature-based, or made with raising operators. Certain vegetables, organic products, grains, nuts, and seeds are not permitted.

About Dr. Sebi

The motivation behind the Dr. Sebi diet originates from local Honduran, Dr. Sebi (genuine name Alfredo Darrington Bowman), who recognizes himself as a botanist, universal healer, and intracellular advisor. The methodology of DrSebi is somewhat fascinating and includes the centering of regular, alkaline, plant-based nourishments, and herbs while avoiding acidic, crossover food sources that can harm the phone. By following the methodology of Alfredo Bowman (otherwise known as Dr. Sebi), you can anticipate bodily fluid develop, which can prompt the advancement of diseases. Dr. Sebi is the author of the USHA Healing Village situated in Honduras, which gives mending, yet additionally shows individuals how to carry on with an alkaline way of life.

Therapeutic experts frequently accept that the DrSebi herb's way of dealing with relieving disease is insufficient because they were instructed to have faith in the drug way to deal with treating patients. This point of view prompted DrSebi and his astonishing home grown mixes showing up on headline news for being sent to the Supreme Court in New York, blaming DrSebi for making bogus cases of restoring individuals and rehearsing prescription without a permit. In any case, numerous individuals have asserted that the DrSebi diet has improved their health altogether with the mixes from DrSebi and that the homegrown way to deal with human recuperating has worked superior to the therapeutic approach to deal with medication. Dr. Sebi's musings about wholesome mixes and homegrown treatment are discovered all through Youtube, instructing, and advance healthy living much after his passing.

Bowman is a motivation to numerous and is a remarkable botanist since he found an approach to recuperate hazardous diseases that have been viewed as severe. He was a cultivator for 40 or more years and cases to recover individuals from AIDS, asthma, cancer, diabetes, dermatitis, epilepsy, fibroids, coronary illness, hypertension, aggravation, lupus, different sclerosis, and sickle cell in addition to other things.

The Dr. Sebi Diet is just a veggie-lover, plant-based diet that limits human-made nourishment and half and halves. The botanist DrSebi diet is tied in with limiting acidity in your nourishments and bodily fluid in your body. Dr. Sebi (otherwise called Alfredo Bowman) accepts that when you do these two things, you make an alkaline domain in your body that makes it intense for the disease to live in. The bodily fluid decreasing alkaline diet from your most loved Dr includes eating from an exclusive nourishing aide and nourishment list that depends on 40+ long periods of research distinguishing non-crossover, alkaline nourishments while additionally enjoying a homegrown embodiment of cell nourishment. Usually, the vast majority get thinner when eating as per the DrSebi plant-based, alkaline diet since they are dispensing with squander, meat, dairy, and prepared nourishments from their food. Frequently individuals join fasting and herbs with the DrSebi diet also to help with purifying, mending a cell or two, and additionally generally speaking prosperity. In these cases, they typically counsel with a specialist or health care proficient.

Nourishing Guide

Adhering to the DrSebi diet long haul isn't that difficult if you can move beyond the initial scarcely any days. The underlying days can be testing; however, as you will, at present, desire sugar. It doesn't help that there are inexpensive food choices all over the place and that most cafés don't have menu things that fit this way of life. Thus, you should become accustomed to setting up a lot of suppers at home. To help with this, we made a recipe book that incorporates an item/course of action that gives all of you of the data you have to eat right, plan out your suppers, and have a great time, delightful recipes that cling to the Dr. Sebi diet.

What Does The Diet Consist of?

The Dr. Sebi diet is a vegetarian, plant-based diet and a specialty rendition of an alkaline diet (Source: National Institute of Health). While following the diet, numerous likewise take herbs to sustain the cell, help cleanse them, and recuperate them of many years of poor eating. Dr. Sebi believes alkaline nourishments to be "electric nourishments" for your battery which are live and crude nourishments that are for the "mending of the country." when all is said in done, DrSebi separates nourishment into six classifications:

- ;• Live
- Raw
- Dead
- Hybrid
- Genetically adjusted
- Drugs

Cultivator Sebi says that you should concentrate on numbers 1 and 2 (live and crude) while avoiding 3 – 6. This incorporates maintaining a strategic distance from seedless organic products, climate-safe yields, for example, corn, and anything with included nutrients or minerals which can be hard for individuals thinking about that there are such a large number of half and a half and hereditarily adjusted (GMO) leafy foods offered in supermarkets as indicated by DrSebi, nourishments that are prescribed for individuals that need to live healthy incorporate ready natural product, non-bland vegetables, crude nuts, and margarine and grains. Verdant greens, quinoa, rye, and Kamut can likewise assume an enormous job in the Dr. Sebi diet. Acidic nourishments including meat, poultry, fish, or items containing yeast, liquor, sugar, iodized salt, or anything that is singed carry negative impacts on the human body.

Supplanting acidic nourishments with electric

alternatives will recuperate you from the negative impacts that acid produces. Following to a great extent, raw diets can appear to be unappetizing to acidic people. Yet, you gradually begin to become accustomed to a raw diet as you cleanse your cells of poisons, prompting the fix of disease. The Vegan Food for the Soul Cookbook improves veggie-lover alkaline living for you! This recipe book incorporates delightful recipes, courses of events, and tips to live healthily.

Limiting acid in nourishments diminishes bodily fluid in the body, which makes an alkaline situation that makes it hard for the disease to shape. Remembering herbs for your purging methodology is far and away superior.

What Is an Acid Alkaline Diet?

Many individuals have been battling to locate the best diet program fit for them. One of the most well-known distortions that these individuals want to get more fit. They neglect to put fundamental accentuation on the best way to be healthy. If you need to know the best diet that is ideal for you, at that point, you better ensure it's healthy and isn't crushing your body.

You need to concede that a diet called the Alkaline diet indeed doesn't have a ton of offer. It's additionally called the alkaline acid diet or the acid-alkaline diet. This is a diet that accentuates eating new products of the soil, tubers, and nuts, and vegetables. The alkaline diet isn't so scary as the name makes it sound, even though it is altogether different from what the vast majority eat. It depends on eating hardly any handled plans or creatures.

The idea is quite straightforward. You should eat that things that you know are useful for your health, for example, vegetables, and new verdant vegetables and you should keep away from things that are awful for you, for example, liquor, yeast, terrible fats, and sugar. The examination is somewhat more intricate than this basic breakdown. Yet, the primary concern is to boost the measure of chemical products of the soil that you eat, just as alkaline squeezes and waters.

It accentuates the 80/20 split of alkaline nourishments to acidic food sources. This is the proportion you should focus on. If it sounds excessively confusing, don't stress since it's not. The vast majority of the nourishments we eat, when they are entirely processed will be either alkaline or acidic. This incorporates fish, grains, meat, shellfish, poultry, salt, and milk produce acid, all healthy in the western diet. While you ought to eat nourishments that are progressively alkaline; for example, new foods are grown from the ground, it doesn't generally play out that way. Therefore we have blood that is somewhat alkaline yet still with normal pH levels somewhere in the range of 7.35 and 7.45.

The theory behind the alkaline diet is that you ought

to eat food that mirrors your body's pH level and be somewhat salty. This is how it was for our progenitors. This is a diet that is inverse to the high fat, high protein, low carb diets that have gotten the "in diets." Most have never known about the alkaline diet or the alkaline acid equalization of the body. Yet, all-encompassing specialists and nutritionists are frequently advocates of this diet since it's accepted this sort of parity is essential to remain healthy and counteract the diseases like cancer. Then again, numerous customary specialists don't have confidence in or support the Alkaline Diet.

For what reason does one choose to go on an alkaline diet? Many accept interminable disease can benefit from outside intervention by an alkaline diet. At present, there isn't a great deal of pertinent information to back this specific diet. Yet, generally simply the nourishments it empowers you to eat are healthy nourishments that are embraced by most specialists. This diet may help individuals who don't feel well when they eat food that is low in carbs or high in protein. It could likewise profit those that have unpleasant lives and who consume such a large number of acidic nourishments. It's always a smart thought to converse with your primary care physician before going on any diet. On the off chance that you have kidney disappointment intense or interminable, you ought not to attempt this diet without your primary care physician's supervision.

The Alkaline Diet

Most likely, you have experienced an alkaline dinner program someplace on the web or in some understanding materials. What is an alkaline diet, and is this diet healthy for you? This diet all began when specialists took a stab at considering the pH level of the body. In an individual's body, the earth can be acidic or alkaline. When the pH level is high, then nature is chemical. In opposite, low pH implies the environment is acidic. The body doesn't have one single pH level; slightly, it can contrast contingent upon the area. The pH level in the stomach is unique about the urinary bladder.

This diet is mainly about eating nourishments which can advance alkaline condition in the body while not eating food sources that elevate acidity to the body. What could be the purpose of this program? To begin, nourishments that can advance an alkaline situation in the body, are viewed as healthy. Instances of these nourishments incorporate vegetables, organic products, soy items, nuts, vegetables, and oats. On the off chance that you have seen, these nourishments are plentiful in protein, nutrients, and minerals.

The other rule of an alkaline diet is to dodge acid nourishments because these are food sources that can make your body in danger for weight gain, heart issues, kidney, and liver diseases. Not many of the numerous acid nourishments incorporate caffeine, food sources with high additives like canned merchandise, soft drinks, fish, meat, liquor, and nourishments with high sugar content. At the point when you then again, the alkaline diet isn't uncommon for everybody, particularly when discussing a healthy diet.

As per specialists, acidic nourishments can diminish the pH of an individual's pee. At the point when the pH is unusually low, kidney stones will appear in general structure. To check this circumstance, an individual needs to expand the pH through eating alkaline-rich nourishments, that basic.

Since an alkaline diet implies keeping away from the liquor and some other nourishments with high acidity, it likewise means that you will diminish the danger of treating diseases related to an unhealthy diet like diabetes, hypertension, and weight. Albeit no careful confirmations can demonstrate, a few scientists have expressed that the alkaline diet can lessen the danger of cancer.

Things to Remember

Altogether, for an alkaline diet to work, you should condition yourself to stick to the diet program. At the point when it expects you to maintain a strategic distance from unhealthy nourishments and drinks, at that point, you better do it. Water treatment is a magnificent elective drink for pop and liquor. Moreover, so you won't make some troublesome memories making sense of which are alkaline and which are acid nourishments; you should make a rundown of every classification.

Maybe you can examine online on what nourishments are wealthy in alkaline and those having high acid substance. Alkaline nourishments are not unreasonably challenging to point because most of the nourishments have a place with vegetables and organic products arrangement.

The Alkaline Diet Myth

The alkaline diet is otherwise called the acid-alkaline diet or the alkaline debris diet. It is based around the possibility that the nourishments you eat dessert a "debris" buildup after they have been utilized. This debris can be acid or alkaline. Defenders of this diet guarantee that specific nourishments can influence the acidity and alkalinity of natural liquids, including pee and blood. On the off chance that you eat nourishments with acidic debris, they make the body acidic. On the off chance that you eat nourishments with alkaline waste, they make the body alkaline.

Acid debris is thought to make you helpless against diseases, for example, cancer, osteoporosis, and muscle squandering, while alkaline waste is viewed as defensive. To ensure you remain alkaline, it is prescribed that you monitor your pee utilizing convenient pH test strips. For the individuals who don't wholly comprehend human physiology and are not sustenance specialists, diet claims like this sound rather persuading. Be that as it may, is it genuinely evident? The accompanying will expose this myth and clear up some disarray concerning the alkaline diet.

On the whole, it is essential to comprehend the significance of pH esteem. Put just; the pH esteem is a proportion of how acidic or alkaline something is. The pH esteem ranges from 0 to 14.

- 0-7 is acidic
- Seven is unbiased
- 7-14 is alkaline

For instance, the stomach is stacked with profoundly acidic hydrochloric acid, pH esteem somewhere in the range of 2 and 3.5. The acidity helps eliminate germs and separate nourishment.

Then again, the human blood is in every case marginally alkaline, with a pH of between the ranges of 7.35 to 7.45. Typically, the body has a few successful components (examined later) to keep the blood pH inside this range. Dropping out of it is intense and can be deadly.

Impacts of Foods on Urine and Blood pH

Nourishments desert an acid or alkaline debris. Acid debris contains phosphate and sulfur. Chemical waste contains calcium, magnesium, and potassium.

Specific nutritional categories are viewed as acidic,

nonpartisan, or alkaline.

- Acidic: Meats, fish, dairy, eggs, grains, and liquor.
- Neutral: Fats, starches, and sugars.
- Alkaline: Fruits, vegetables, nuts, and vegetables.

Urine pH

Nourishments you eat change the pH of your pee. If you have a green smoothie for breakfast, your pee, in a couple of hours, will be more alkaline than if you had bacon and eggs. For somebody on an alkaline diet, pee pH can be effectively checked and may even give moment delight. Sadly, pee pH is neither a decent pointer of the general pH of the body, nor is it a suitable marker of public health.

Blood pH

Nourishments you eat don't change your blood pH. At the point when you eat something with acid debris like protein, the acids created are immediately killed by bicarbonate particles in the blood. This response produces carbon dioxide, which is breathed out through the lungs, and salts, which are discharged by the kidneys in your pee. During the procedure of discharge, the kidneys produce new bicarbonate particles, which are come back to the blood to supplant the bicarbonate that was at first used to kill the acid. This makes a reasonable cycle wherein the body can keep up the pH of the blood inside a tight range.

In this way, as long as your kidneys are working typically, your blood pH won't be impacted by the nourishments you eat, regardless of whether they are acidic or alkaline. The case that eating alkaline nourishments will make your body or blood pH progressively alkaline isn't valid.

Acidic Diet And Cancer

The individuals who advocate an alkaline diet guarantee that it can fix cancer since cancer can just develop in an acidic domain. By eating an alkaline diet, cancer cells can't develop; however, bite the dust. This speculation is exceptionally defective. Cancer is flawlessly equipped for developing in an alkaline situation. Cancer develops in healthy body tissue, which has a somewhat alkaline pH of 7.4. Numerous analyses have affirmed this by effectively developing cancer cells in an alkaline domain.

Be that as it may, cancer cells do become quicker with acidity. When a tumor begins to create, it makes its very own acidic condition by separating glucose and decreasing flow. Along these lines, it isn't the acidic condition that causes cancer, yet cancer that causes the acidic disease. Significantly all the more fascinating is a recent report by the National Cancer Institute, which utilizes nutrient C (ascorbic acid) to treat cancer. They found that by directing pharmacologic portions intravenously, ascorbic acid effectively murdered cancer cells without hurting healthy cells. This is another case of cancer cells being powerless against acidity, instead of alkalinity.

To put it plainly, there is no logical connection between eating an acidic diet and cancer. Cancer cells can develop in both acidic and alkaline conditions.

Acidic Diet And Osteoporosis

Osteoporosis is a progressive bone disease described by a decline in bone mineral substance, prompting brought down the bone thickness and quality and greater danger of a messed up bone. Advocates of the alkaline diet accept that to keep up a steady blood pH, the body takes alkaline minerals like calcium from the unresolved issues the acids from acidic food. As examined over, this is in no way, shape, or form genuine. The kidneys and the respiratory framework are answerable for managing blood pH, not the bones.

Numerous examinations have indicated that expanding creature protein admission is sure for bone digestion as it builds calcium maintenance and actuates IGF-1 (insulin-like development factor-1) that animates bone recovery. In this manner, the speculation that an acidic diet causes bone loss isn't upheld by science.

Acidic Diet And Muscle Wasting

Backers of the alkaline diet accept that to dispense with overabundance acid brought about by acidic food, the kidneys will take amino acids (building squares of protein) from muscle tissues, prompting muscle loss. The proposed system is like the one causing osteoporosis. As examined, blood pH is controlled by the kidneys and the lungs, not the muscles. Thus, acidic nourishments like meats, dairy, and eggs don't cause muscle loss. Indeed, they are complete dietary proteins that will bolster muscle fix and help anticipate muscle squandering.

What Did Our Ancestors Eat?

Various investigations have inspected whether our pre-farming predecessors ate net acidic or net alkaline diets. Interestingly, they found that about portion of the tracker gatherers ate net acid-framing foods, while the other half ate profit alkaline-shaping diets. Acid-framing meals were progressively regular as individuals moved further north of the equator. The less approachable the earth, the more creature proteins they ate. In progressively tropical conditions where foods grown from the ground were plenteous, their diet turned out to be increasingly alkaline.

From a developmental point of view, the theory that acidic or protein-rich diets cause diseases like cancer, osteoporosis, and muscle loss isn't substantial. Half of the tracker gatherers were eating net acid-shaping foods, yet, they had no proof of such degenerative diseases. There must be nobody size-fits-all diet that works for everybody, which is the reason Metabolic Typing is so useful in deciding your ideal menu. Because of our genetic changes, a few people will profit from an acidic diet, around an alkaline diet, and some in the middle. In this manner, the maxim: short time's nourishment can be another man's toxin.

The facts confirm that numerous individuals who have changed to an alkaline diet see massive health enhancements. In any case, do remember that different reasons might be grinding away:

• Most of us don't eat enough vegetables and natural products. As indicated by the Center for Disease and Prevention, just 9% of Americans eat enough vegetables and 13% enough natural products. If you change to an alkaline diet, you are consequently eating more vegetables and organic products. They are wealthy in phytochemicals, cancer prevention agents, and fiber, which are essential to excellent health. At the point when you eat more vegetables and natural products, you are presumably eating less handled nourishments as well.

• Eating less dairy and eggs will profit the individuals who are lactose-bigoted or have a nourishment affectability to eggs, which is relatively healthy among the all-inclusive community.

Eating fewer grains will profit the individuals who are gluten-delicate or have broken gut or an immune system disease.

Alkaline Water

One final point worth referencing is that numerous individuals accept that drinking alkaline water (pH of 9.5 versus pure water's pH of 7.0.) is healthier dependent on comparable thinking as the alkaline diet. At any rate, it isn't valid. Water that is too alkaline can be contrary to your health and lead to wholesome disequilibrium.

On the off chance that you drink alkaline water regularly, it will kill your stomach acid and raise the alkalinity of your stomach. After some time, it will impede your capacity to process nourishment and assimilate supplements and minerals. With less acidity in the stomach, it will likewise open the entryway for microscopic organisms and parasites to get into your small digestive system. Most importantly, alkaline water isn't a response to excellent health. Try not to be tricked by showcasing contrivances. Instead, put resources into a decent water filtration framework for your home. Clean, separated water is as yet the best water for your body.

Straightforward With an Alkaline Diet

At the point when you decide to eat an alkaline diet,

you are eating nourishments that are fundamentally the same as what man was intended to eat. If you take a gander at what our progenitors ate, you will discover a diet wealthy in new natural products, vegetables, vegetables, nuts, and fish. Shockingly, man's diet today is much of the time loaded with nourishments that are high in unhealthy fats, salt, cholesterol, and acidifying food sources.

How Our Diet Changed

Albeit a few people believe that man's diet changed as of late, the move from or to an excellent extent alkaline diet to an acid diet started a considerable number of years back. Our unique diet comprised of scavenged natural products, nuts, and vegetables, alongside whatever meat could be gotten. When man began to develop his very own nourishment, things began to change. Grains turned into a well-known diet decision, particularly after the advancement of stone instruments. When creatures were trained, there were dairy items added to the diet, alongside an extra measure of meat. Salt started to be included, alongside sugar. The final product was a diet that was still a lot healthier than what numerous individuals eat today. However, the move from alkaline to acid had started.

Late Dietary Changes

It's a well-known fact that our advanced diet

comprises of numerous nourishments which are not healthy for us. An excessive amount of shoddy nourishment and "inexpensive food" has diminished the nature of our menu. Heftiness has become the standard and alongside it a higher rate of diseases, for example, diabetes, coronary disease, and cancer. On the off chance that you need to improve your health and lessen the danger of numerous diseases, an alkaline diet can help recover your body to nuts and bolts.

At the point when nourishments are eaten and processed, they produce either an acidifying or alkalizing impact inside the body. A few people get confounded because the real pH of the nourishment itself doesn't have anything to do with the effects of the food once it is processed. At the point when progressively alkaline nourishments are devoured, the body can turn out to be marginally alkaline rather than acid. Preferably, the blood pH level ought to be somewhere in the range of 7.35 and 7.45. Nourishments, for example, organic citrus products, soy items, homemade leafy foods, wild rice, almonds, and regular sugars, for instance, Stevia are generally significant alkaline nourishment decisions.

Advantages of an Alkaline Diet

There are numerous advantages to moving your eating designs from acid to alkaline. At the point when the body is kept somewhat alkaline, it is less helpless to disease. It's simpler to shed pounds or keep up a healthy weight level on an alkaline diet. A great many people experience an expansion in their energy level, just as a decreasing of uneasiness and fractiousness once they start eating increasingly caustic nourishments. Mucous creation is diminished, and the nasal clog is decreased, making it simpler to breathe. Hypersensitivities are much of the time mitigated because of an alkaline diet. The body is additionally less helpless to diseases, for example, cancer and diabetes. A great many people find that they simply feel good, with an expanded feeling of health and prosperity, when they endeavor to hold fast to an alkaline diet.

Picking Alkaline Diets Is The Only Way To Live A Healthy Lifestyle

The low carbohydrate and high protein diets doing the rounds nowadays are a solicitation to poor health. All competitors realize that if a fit body is to be kept up, one should avoid such diets. In addition to the fact that they result in extreme weariness are where weight the executives are concerned. Picking alkaline foods is the best way to carry on with a healthy life just as shed those additional pounds.

Alkaline diets expect one to pursue a way of direct life inverse of the high protein low carb diets. The high protein diets leave the individual tailing it exhausted and tired. It is for the individuals who have a dormant existence and need to shed some weight. In any case, the weight that is lost returns on when one stops the diet. With alkaline foods, this isn't the situation. The menus can be joined into one's lifestyle, and inside days the outcomes start to show. They expect one to eat around 80 % alkalizing nourishments to keep up the alkaline ph. of the body to 7.4. High protein diets will, in general, make the ph. of the body acidic instead of its standard alkaline tilt at the point when the body ph. becomes acidic. It pulls in all sicknesses and exhausts one of energy — an acidic ph.

Additionally brings about quick degeneration of the human body cells. That prompts an abbreviated life. One should avoid these accident diets and take a gander at accomplishing health and energy by following alkaline foods.

Alkaline diets lead to body ph. It is keeping up its chemical nature. The different body capacities are completed quickly, and the insusceptible arrangement of the body remains solid. Under these conditions, one feels enthusiastic rather than feeling exhausted. Additionally, the weight shed like this stays off, and in particular, the body doesn't fall debilitated. As such, they help repulse diseases instead of high protein diets, which appear to pull in them. These plans are likewise generally excellent for those experiencing interminable diseases like joint pain, cancer, headaches, sinusitis, and osteoporosis. Following such a system while taking prescription helps fend these diseases off from the root.

Alkaline diets generally comprise of foods grown from the ground. One should attempt to expend green vegetables and sweet natural products with the goal that they make up around 70 to 80 percent of their all-out nourishment admission. Lemons and melons ought to likewise be eaten. Almonds, nectar, and olive oil are additionally high on the rundown of nourishments to be expended for following alkaline diets. Meats and fats ought to stay away from. All nourishments that are acidifying like espresso, liquor, pork, and even certain vegetables like cooked spinach ought not to shape over 20% of one's diet. Alkaline water is additionally an unquestionable requirement for everybody needing to improve their diet. At any rate, 6 to 8 glasses of alkaline water can do wonders for your body purifying. Prepared nourishment is all acidic and high on weight picking up substances, thus ought to be kept away from. Drinks like soft drinks are profoundly acidic and ought not to be expended by any stretch of the imagination. It takes 32 glasses of water to adjust one glass of pop. Alkaline diets are for everybody. Every last one of us should quit manhandling our bodies and take a gander at a healthy and long life by making alkaline diets a piece of our way of life.

The Alkaline Diet - What Can I Eat on It?

The Alkaline Diet is otherwise called the Alkaline Ash Diet, Alkaline Acid Diet, or the Acid Alkaline Diet. Specialists, for example, Robert O. Youthful, N.D. are supporting this diet, and accept nourishment can be delegated alkaline, acid, or nonpartisan as per pH. By and large, the menu comprises of eating particular citrus, other low sugar organic products, vegetables, tubers, nuts, and vegetables. Grains, dairy items, meat, sugar, liquor, caffeine, and organisms like mushrooms are to be maintained a strategic distance from. By expending such a diet, it is said that the body keeps up a pH of somewhere in the range of 7.35 and 7.45 (7.00 is impartial on the pH scale while beneath 7.00 is acidic).

Diet And Disease

There is some proof that such a diet is useful in anticipating osteoporosis and other bone health issues. In any case, the evidence isn't substantial in supporting the instances that an alkaline diet may forestall or help lighten conditions, for example, cancer, weakness, heftiness, or sensitivities. There is, in any case, some proof that cancer cells develop all the more rapidly in an acidic situation in a research center setting. In this manner, an individual with an inclination to or who experiences this disease might need to research the impacts an alkaline diet has on the body.

Considering the mind-boggling ascend in a large

number of these sorts of diseases, it is anything but difficult to think about whether they are brought about by the general state of an individual's interior body condition. A more extensive and all the more deductively fiery assessment of the Alkaline Diet is altogether. Be that as it may, such logical examination might be polluted from the earliest starting point by partiality instigated in a pharmaceutical-based health care delivery framework.

The theory behind the Alkaline Diet isn't broadly acknowledged by the therapeutic network, which might be one reason cancer, diabetes, and any number of other awful diseases are at pandemic levels. The Alkaline Diet, when joined with a physically dynamic, low-pressure way of life, surely merits more consideration from established researchers if they can keep their predisposition under control.

It would be generally easy to check whether specific conditions, for example, glucose, pulse, cholesterol tally, and an individual's weight standardize when (and if) their blood pH falls into the ideal range. These indications happen together so regularly that the medicinal network has started calling it Syndrome X. If this syndrome is so healthy and the convention for logical assessment so necessary, for what reason is the Alkaline Diet still, for example, riddle about whether it is valuable or not?

It might be because there is no cash to be produced using prescribing a particular diet. Pharmaceutical organizations test new drugs because there is a benefit to be made if the drug makes it advertise. Be that as it may, there is no benefit in dietary suggestions. In this way, such research would tumble to the colleges and administrative organizations to direct. The idea that the more significant part of those analysts likewise fills in as experts for the pharmaceutical business may effectively spoil their eagerness and discoveries.

Great Healthy Food

All in all, what are you expected to eat? It is prescribed that you maintain a strategic distance from "acidic" nourishments, for example, sugar, red meat, shellfish, eggs, dairy, prepared, and other refined food sources, most grains including refined grains, fake sugars, liquor, caffeine, chocolate, and soft drink. You ought to devour crude products of the soil that have a high chlorophyll substance, for example, verdant green vegetables.

The brassica group of vegetables (otherwise called crucifers) are very much spoken to on the Alkaline Diet and include:

- Broccoli
- Brussels grows
- Cabbage

- Cauliflower
- Turnips
- Collard greens
- Kale
- Kohlrabi
- Bok Choi
- Mustard Greens

Other crude vegetables to take a stab at your alkaline diet are:

- Avocado
- Tomato
- Red Beets
- Carrots
- Lima Beans
- Red and dark radishes
- Rutabaga
- Eggplant
- Asparagus
- Artichoke
- Lettuce
- Endive

- Cucumber
- Celery
- Peppers
- Zucchini
- Squash
- Spinach
- Peas
- Parsnips
- Onions

Healthy Fruit

The best organic product to devour on the alkaline diet incorporates:

- Unripe bananas
- Sour fruits
- Fresh coconut
- Figs (either crude or dried)
- Fresh lemon
- Lime

Regardless of whether the Alkaline Diet is as useful for forestalling disease as its advocate's guarantee should hold back to be seen. Be that as it may, following the alkaline diet surely will keep you inside the parameters of what most other restorative experts and associations have been professing to be a healthy diet for some, numerous years.

The Theory of the Alkaline Diet

To keep your body crisp and liberated from diseases, you need to eat the correct nourishment called an alkaline diet or acid-alkaline diet. Essentially it is a theory that when we eat or devour food, after a few procedures like processing, digestion, and others, it leaves a chemical buildup or acid buildup, which decides the acid-alkaline nature of our body.

Alkaline diet theory depends on the way that the pH of our body is somewhat salty, which is from 7.35 to 7.45 (in certain writings, it is 7.36 to 7.44). Our diet ought to speak to this parity. An aggravation in this equalization will cause some severe issues in the body. The idea of fluid, whether acidic or alkaline, is dictated by the pH scale. It ranges from 0 (in number acid) to 14 (in number alkaline). 7 is the neutral point on pH as that of water. A pH underneath 7 shows acid things, as we go down, getting solid acidic, and pH over seven speaks to alkaline items, power expanding as we go up to 14.

Therapeutic investigation of pretty much every sort has alkaline diet roots even though this theory does not recognize by traditional medicinal social orders. Diets that contain 60% alkalinity ought to be utilized to keep up the parity of the body. One needs to use profoundly alkaline foods (80%) is the equalization of his/her body is upset by the broad utilization of meat, eggs, cream, and other acidic nourishments.

Vegetables, low-fat natural products, nuts, tubers, crisp citrus, and different things ought to be favored when discussing alkaline diets. To expand alkalinity in the body, organic products can be utilized as a decent source as, for the most part, natural products are wealthy in alkaline. Not many numbers of natural products are acidic. When eating natural products, for this reason, don't eat canned, or sugared or safeguarded organic products, since they become exceptionally acidic when saved because of the utilization of various synthetic compounds.

Vegetables are energetically prescribed in alkaline diet theory as they are an excellent wellspring of making the body alkaline. You will feel shortcoming as opposed to control in your body if the meat you are eating to pick up energy becomes an acid framing operator in your body, as ordinary specialists don't trust in eating vegetables could be valuable and continue eating meat for strength.

Vegetables, particularly green vegetables, are generally excellent wellspring of alkaline creation, and you can utilize them cooked. However, vegetables like carrot, cauliflower, tomatoes, and others are being used whenever you need without cooking. They are scrumptious and furnish you with heaps of minerals. Minerals like calcium, potassium, and magnesium are the genuine wellspring of alkaline debris and are excellent for the development and working of the body. Our body is abandoned acidic to marginally soluble when these minerals respond with the acid present in our collection.

High Alkaline Diet - Tips on How to Maintain a Healthy Body by Having an Alkaline Diet

A considerable lot of us, without a doubt, have found out about a high alkaline diet. This sort of food has been demonstrated as compelling and useful. You must have this sort of nutrition if you need to help your resistant framework, bringing about a healthy way of life. An alkaline diet is a sort of eating where you ought to have the option to devour substantially more alkaline nourishments as opposed to acid food sources. The alkaline to acid admission proportion must be 4:1. Alkaline nourishments are anything but difficult to have, and they are known to give more advantages to us.

Acid nourishments, then again, are food sources that we know are awful for our health. These incorporate handled nourishments, red meat, dairy items, and others. Nourishments containing omega-six fats are terrible for our health, and they are viewed as acidic. This incorporates corn oil, sunflower oil, and soybean oil. We realize that getting fats from meats is genuinely not great. They cause hypertension and elevated cholesterol level. Fats and carbohydrates, when taken in a considerable sum, are wrong. Carbohydrates are separated into sugar upon digestion. At the point when we eat nourishments with a lot of carbs, and we don't get dynamic, the sugar will, at that point, be put away as fats.

These fats are the guilty parties to carrying on with an unhealthy way of life. They cause such a large number of diseases and obesity. Numerous Western individuals are having issues with unnecessary weight gain. This is an impact of them having increasingly acid nourishments joined in their diets.

How might we keep up a healthy body?
Eat all the more new products of the soil.

We realize that leafy foods are beneficial for us. The majority of them are viewed as alkaline nourishments. Just a few are most certainly not. Indeed, even those products of the soil that are acid in their normal state are considered as alkaline nourishments. Among them are lemons, lime, and grapefruits.

Alkaline nourishments are those that, when used by the body, produce caustic debris and kill acid debris inside the body. A high alkaline diet is key to not bargaining our health. The high acidity makes our bones and different joints debilitate because the acid removes the calcium and various supplements for balance.

In this way, we ought to have a high admission of alkaline framing nourishments. If we did, our health would be reestablished.

Exercise routinely.

Day by day practice indeed encourages an individual to get stimulated, and it helps the psyche and body to work well. It additionally helps in the best possible oxygen delivery all through our body framework. It likewise helps in legitimate processing and advances unique dietary patterns.

Drink enough water. It is much improved if you drink alkaline water.

Notwithstanding eating a high alkaline diet, we ought to likewise drink a lot of water. In any case, we should realize that it is smarter to have our water alkalized. This is the thing that we call alkaline water. It is known to be useful for our health.

Attempt An Alkaline Diet - Eating Alkaline Foods

To become healthy, you need to think fit, and this is the reason numerous individuals nowadays are going to alkaline nourishment diets. This is fantastic for both your health and your body. Individuals on this diet had asserted they feel great as well as have more energy and improved assimilation and considerably less emotional episodes than before they began.

An alkaline diet is mostly eating alkaline nourishments. The establishment of this diet is vegan. To get the best from this diet, we will give you some direction beneath.

• Vegetables would be ostensibly the most basic nourishment around. Simple to purchase and simple to plan.

• Try to pick entire grain nourishments as opposed to prepared ones because handled items don't have the equivalent wholesome substance.

• Some acidic nourishments, for example, limes, lemons, and grapefruits, go-to alkaline after processing, so are valuable for enhancing.

• Other acidic nourishments additionally ready to be utilized in this diet are espresso, cola, and broccoli, artichoke, asparagus, beetroot, spinach, and cauliflower.

• Avocado, celery, garlic, ginger, onions, pumpkin are perfect vegetables to incorporate.

• Tomatoes, pears, papayas, mango, apricots, and apples can be incorporated.

• Nuts to utilize are sunflower seeds, almonds, and pecans.

• Oats, dark colored rice, and almond and darker rice drain just as coconut and coconut water can likewise be utilized.

What to Avoid

• Red meat, poultry, dairy items, and bubbly drinks are the nourishments that are the hardest to process. Your kidneys need to take minerals, which are crucial for the body, similar to calcium and magnesium, from the bones to break up the acid in these nourishments.

It is not necessarily the case that little amounts of the above can't be utilized to enhance and change up your dinners. You will before long acknowledge precisely what you can and can't use, as your body will before long let you know.

Move towards this alkaline diet continuously. On the off chance that you eat a ton of meat or love dairy nourishments like cheddar, it might be ideal to attempt an alkaline diet supper three times each week, to begin with, so your body doesn't go into stun. Any diet must be drawn nearer delicately, and once your body acknowledges the new nourishments being offered, it will thank you by looking and feeling better.

As a rule, the pH of alkaline in our blood is estimated from 7.35 to 7.45, and the degree of acid is from 1.0 to 9.0. Changing your way of life by receiving this alkaline diet could make you feel much healthier than you do now.

Healthiest Alkaline Diet Foods

Have you ever known about alkaline diet nourishments? If not, it's about time that you do. Work pressure, homemaking, keeping up close to home, and expert relations are negatively affecting everybody's nourishment propensities, bringing about over 70% of the present age experiencing acidity and indigestion. Each third individual is by all accounts whining of gastric issues, heartburn, and acid reflux. The entirety of this is because of the lopsidedness in the acid-alkaline pH of nourishments that expended nowadays, where you just snatch something and hurry to work. Quick nourishments, soft drinks, and so forth are being consumed left, right, and focus by a young age, therefore offering to ascend to lack in minerals, nutrients, and sustenance.

Alkaline diets have been seen as exceptionally gainful for ideal health. You can keep persistent diseases, for example, acidity, osteoporosis, and summed up shortcoming at a manageable distance with nourishments wealthy in alkaline substance. Alkaline nourishments are significant since the pH of human blood is marginally progressively alkaline. This makes it vital that we have a higher amount of alkaline pH than acidic substances in the body.

What are the advantages of Alkaline Diets?

Alkaline diet nourishments have plenty of advantages, for example,

- Improved obstruction
- Vibrant disposition
- Increased Alertness
- Strong teeth and Bones
- Easy Digestion

Alkaline diet nourishments are crucial to keeping up the pH levels of blood at an ideal of 7. Alkaline nourishments are, for the most part, vegan food sources comprising of new nourishments and vegetables.

Recorded here are the best ten healthiest alkaline nourishments for dietary advantages:

1. Spinach and Greens - Spinach has been found to contain the most extreme positions and is exceptionally caustic. It very well may be devoured crude or cooked with equivalent impact. Other verdant green vegetables, for example, lettuce, fenugreek leaves, basil, and so on likewise, are amazingly high as alkaline nourishments. They additionally contain many minerals and nutrients as an extra bit of leeway.

2. Cucumber - Raw cucumber isn't just a zero-calorie vegetable; it is profoundly alkaline when expended crude. It is heavenly and contains a large group of dietary advantages. Cucumber improves in general absorption and keeps your skin new and gleaming. It contains healthy alkaline water that aids in flushing out undesirable squanders from the body.

3. Banana - Banana can be viewed in general nourishment due to its various dietary favorable circumstances. It gives moment energy and is gigantically alkaline. Truth be told, if you are experiencing severe acidic issues, a banana diet can do some fantastic things in decreasing the consuming sensation and heartburn astoundingly. Bananas have fresh sugar content and can be devoured by anybody independent of his health condition.

4. Celery - Celery is heavenly alkaline nourishment that can help you gigantically in keeping your pH levels at the ordinary scope of 7. At the point when half-cooked, it gives the most significant health benefit and can be eaten as a new plate of mixed greens as well.

5. Broccoli - Broccoli is one of the most nutritious and alkaline nourishments that has substantiated itself on numerous occasions. It is effectively edible and is a rich wellspring of significant minerals, for example, carotene and calcium. These minerals help in improving insusceptibility and battle diseases in an unusual way.

6. Avocado - This miracle organic product is a rich wellspring of alkaline nourishment and has a general advantage in keeping up excellent health. Avocado improves your hemoglobin content and is incredibly gainful in reestablishing commonality in a disease influenced body.

7. Capsicum - Capsicum, otherwise called ringer

pepper, is a rich enemy of oxidant and can be valuable, whether eaten cooked or crude. It isn't just of high alkaline and dietary benefit, it is additionally delectable and adds taste to any dishes that are set up with capsicum for the season.

8. Potato Skin - Although potato is seen as acidic, potato skin is exceptionally wealthy in alkaline substance. Crude potato juice is seen as valuable in diminishing the acidic content in the stomach.

9. Soybeans - Soybeans and soy milk are extraordinarily alkaline and can be utilized as dietary alkaline nourishments.

10. Cold Milk - Cold milk is found to have high alkaline substance and is regularly prescribed to battle indigestion and acid reflux issue.

Alkaline diet nourishments are getting exceptionally well known among health cognizant people who have understood their incredible advantages and high dietary benefit. In addition to the fact that they help you advance your pH level, however, they likewise improve your general health and assist you with acquiring a sans disease life.

Alkaline Diet For Top Energy

It is safe to say that you are inadequate about energy? Do you want to change your diet for weight loss or some other explanation at all? There are a few diets that are bad for you and some that are beneficial for you. You have to know the distinction, and here it the alkaline diet outline. This sort of diet is one that urges you to eat nourishments that produce an alkaline quality and the blood, and this is the thing that enables our energy to level and enables your body to turn out to be progressively healthy.

The nourishments that help you with regards to the alkaline level in your body are lemons, limes, raw spinach, almonds, alkaline water, avocado, organic products, melons, carrots, lima beans, and numerous other characteristic nourishments. It is effortless to discover a rundown that is a couple of pages of alkaline nourishments. The quickest method to begin your new diet is to start with water. Include three liters of salty water to your diet every day, and you will be en route to excellent food and more energy. Channel your pool with a decent channel and include a cut of lime or lemon into the water to make it alkaline.

The one thing you need to comprehend is that on the off chance that you choose to pursue the alkaline diet, at that point, you have to ensure you keep on having an equalization in your diet. Despite everything, you need meats, dairy, and different nourishments that are not viewed as alkaline. They have supplements that you need in your body to help assemble your resistant framework and your muscles.

Alkaline Diet Secrets - Discover the Secrets of the Alkaline Diet

Have you been searching for an incredible diet to assist you with getting more fit, become healthier, and gain energy? There are numerous decisions about foods, and that is the thing that makes it hard. Nonetheless, there is one diet called the alkaline diet. It is one that will assist you in picking up energy and live healthier. It will likewise enable your body to come back to your optimal weight for your stature. Here are the insider facts of the alkaline diet.

To begin with, you will manage the ph. Level of your body. Essentially, this is the harmony between the acid and the alkaline in your body. The perfect level is 7.4, and you can accomplish this by eating a specific way and drinking a particular way. There is parity to this diet that is fundamental, and you have to comprehend certain things on the off chance that you need to build your energy level and get healthier.

Second, the parity is critical to comprehend. You don't pick up anything by being at a higher ph than what you need. You need to understand that when you buy a manual for this diet, it will discuss the stricter feeling of the menu being that you can't eat creature fragile living creature, and it will instruct you to quit devouring dairy items. This isn't the ideal approach to utilize this diet. You need to keep up a parity because your body needs the things that creatures fragile living creatures and dairy items contain. These nourishments assist us with working up a resistance to specific microbes and help us with warding off ailment.

You need to comprehend that the alkaline diet is incredible for energy, and you can add a little change to your diet to truly support your chemical level. You should simply channel your water and include a cut of lemon or lime to it to make it alkaline. This change alone and 3 liters of this water a day will give you energy, and this is the mystery of the alkaline diet that is ideal.

Alkaline Diet: Acidic And Alkaline Foods

Gastric hyperacidity is one of the most well-known ailments. Besides, metabolic acidosis is said to be the premise of all disease since it is straightforwardly identified with different kidney issues, diabetes, ulcer, and numerous other interior diseases. Subsequently, the motivation behind the alkaline diet is to carry the pH to ordinary and to assist individuals with getting in shape, not through a caloric shortfall, however, by supplanting some other acidic nourishments with alkaline food sources.

The alkaline diet is a cutting edge one that was conceived from the craving/requirement for individuals to treat hyper gastric acidity and anticipate or defer as a lot of issues brought about by acidosis. Alkaline Diet plan includes making compound nourishment as pursues:

a) 75% alkaline nourishments, which have a pH more prominent than 7.4, as near 8;

b) 25% acidic nourishments;

What is the contrast between acidic nourishments and those for the alkaline diet?

As far as a concoction, acidic nourishments are soaked with hydrogen particles, while the alkaline has a synthetic structure that permits the assimilation of hydrogen particles.

Regularly, the inner pH (of blood) is 7.38 to 7, 52. It is indispensable that the pH doesn't drop beneath 7, as this may prompt evaluation IV extreme lethargies and even pass off the patient. Likewise, the blood doesn't must have an essential character, however just marginally alkaline; generally, there is the danger of automatic muscle withdrawals, amazingly groundbreaking and agonizing.

Which nourishments are alkaline, and which are acidic?

In acidic nourishment classification, there are on the whole conventional food sources, soft drinks, cakes, and obviously, mixed refreshments. Chicken, meat, turkey, pasta, refined oil, pickles (extremely acidic!), all treats, and all subordinates of the above items have a generally high acidity, whose worth may rise or fall in relying upon the method of planning.

In the alkaline diet nourishments class we have:

a) Curds, cucumbers and lettuce, avocado and every one of the vegetables and eatable plants wealthy in chlorophyll;

b) Soya milk, soya pieces, coconut, lemon, millet, beans, and buckwheat;

c) Sea buckthorn;

d) Cold squeezed oil of any sort;

Alkaline water is imperative for alkaline diet!

For the individuals who can't keep up the prescribed rate in the diet (75% alkaline nourishments and 25% acidic nourishments), it is prescribed to supplant drinks with alkaline water. Any water that has a pH more noteworthy than 7.7 is viewed as alkaline water and can be devoured in enormous amounts. The danger of blood pH to increment to essential qualities is low, 2.5-3 liters of alkaline water a day should assist anybody with maintaining its ideal health and consistently help detoxify the body and cleaning of free radicals.

Smoking is restricted!

Smoking is a propensity that develops especially acidity in the body, which happens when we drink liquor as well. Accordingly is prescribed that these exercises be limited or killed from your day by day schedule with the goal that the body gets all opportunities to stay healthy and clean. Subsequently, smoking is carefully denied in the alkaline diet.

Where Can I Find Alkaline Diet Recipes?

When you initially find the alkaline diet and its numerous advantages - from incredible degrees of energy and imperativeness to its enemy of maturing properties, extraordinary processing, disease aversion, and a general elevate in health - the usual inquiry is "The place would I be able to discover alkaline diet recipes?" The reviving answer is that numerous recipes and suppers that you know and appreciate can be made progressively alkaline by making some necessary substitutions of nourishments that are alkaline.

Following the alkaline diet implies swapping acidic nourishments like meat, dairy, refined sugars and fats, and other handled food sources for alkaline nourishments, for example, vegetables, verdant greens, a few products of the soil and seeds. So for instance, you can make an alkaline form of spaghetti Bolognese by swapping the minced hamburger for darker lentils, swapping the container of handled Bolognese tomato sauce for a home-made adaptation containing tomatoes, herbs and flavors, some flax oil, onions and a couple of other natural, characteristic fixings mixed and swapping the durum wheat spaghetti for crude corvette noodles made with a vegetable practice.

Another unique alkaline diet recipe that is so great it's difficult to trust it's healthy for you is alkaline banana dessert: You mainly take a lot of over-ready bananas, strip them, cut them up into pieces and freeze them. At that point when you need to eat the dessert, take ten or so of the solidified pieces, mix them in your rapid blender with a little coconut or almond milk and a teaspoon of mica (a calciferous root vegetable super-nourishment that preferences a little malt-like) on the off chance that you wish. You could likewise include some vanilla concentrate or lucuma powder (custard-tasting super nourishment) to make it progressively 'rich.' Straightforward, healthy, delightful! It's genuinely challenging to accept that this frozen yogurt recipe has no dairy in it, and the consistency is much the same as an appropriate dessert.

An inquiry that is posed to a ton is whether organic products are alkaline. The straightforward answer is that it depends: insofar as natural products are eaten alone, before some other more slow processing nourishments and with regards to a general vegetable-based diet, at that point, they supplement this and help to alkalize your body. If they have not consolidated appropriately, at that point, they can age and cause acidification. So it's excellent to advise yourself about ideal nourishment consolidating conventions.

A decent dependable guideline for making recipes alkaline is to keep them as natural as could be allowed - crude, regular fixings are ideal - and by subbing meat and dairy items for vegetables and beans, heartbeats and nuts and seeds. Some straightforward swaps you can undoubtedly make alkalize your diet and body: Coconut milk for dairy milk; steamed vegetables for rice, pasta, and bread; beats for meat; organic products for refined sugar items; water and natural teas for espresso, pop, and liquor.

CHAPTER TWO
BENEFITS OF THE ALKALINE DIET

Human Body Design and Alkaline Diet

The human body is, somewhat, alkaline by structure. By keeping up it salty, we enable it to run at a perfect level. By and by, a massive number of responses of our digestion yield acidic squanders as final results. At the point when we expend an unreasonable measure of acid-delivering nourishments and insufficient alkaline-shaping nourishments, we disturb the body acid inebriation. On the off chance that we let these acid-squanders develop all through the body, a turmoil known as acidosis creates after some time.

Acidosis will continuously cripple our body's indispensable capacities, on the off chance that we don't rapidly take therapeutic activities. Acidosis, or body over-acidity, is, in truth, one of the primary sources of human maturing. It makes our body exceptionally helpless against the arrangement of the savage degenerative interminable diseases, for example, diabetes, cancer, joint pain, just as heart diseases.

Thus, the most significant test we people need to face to ensure our lives is really to locate the correct method to diminish the creation and to boost the end of the body acidic squander. To keep away from acidosis and the age-related diseases, and to keep running at its most elevated level conceivable, our body needs a healthy way of life. This way of life ought to incorporate ordinary activities, fair sustenance, a clean physical condition, and a method for living that brings the most minimal pressure conceivable. A healthy way of life enables our body to keep its acid waste substance at the most reduced level understandable.

The alkaline diet, otherwise called the pH wonder diet, appears to fit the best of the structure of the human body. This is predominantly because it kills the acid squanders and permits flushing them out from the body. Individuals should take a gander at alkaline diet as general dietary limits for people to comply with. The people who have specific health issues and exceptional medicinal foods may better oblige those diets to soluble diet limits.

Alkaline Diet Benefits for Diabetics

The supernatural occurrence of an alkaline diet will help improve the general health of the people experiencing diabetes. As it accomplishes for other individuals, the alkaline diet will help support their body physiology and digestion, just as their insusceptible framework. This diet will enable people with diabetes to have superior control of their glucose. It is likewise going to help not only in diminishing their weight gain and the dangers of cardiovascular diseases, yet in addition to keeping their cholesterol level low.

The alkaline diet permits a superior administration of diabetes and, accordingly, it assists people with diabetes with staying away from all the more effectively the degenerative diseases associated with their condition. So by following an alkaline diet, in spite of their health circumstances, people with diabetes can, simultaneously, live healthier and expand their future significantly.

Diabetics Acid-Alkaline Food Chart

As a rule, individuals who need to pursue an alkaline diet need to choose their day by day nourishment things from an 'Acid-Alkaline Foods Chart.' We as of late distributed a 'Diabetics Acid-Alkaline Food Chart.' The utilization of this particular outline enables people with diabetes to fit in with both the alkaline diet rule and the glycemic list rule. The alkaline diet rule sets wholesome general rules. As per this diet plan, our day by day nourishment admission ought to be made out of at least 80 percent of alkaline-framing nourishments, and of close to 20 percent of acidifying nourishment items. Moreover, the diet features that the more alkaline a nourishment thing is, the better it is really. Then again, the all the more acidifying a nourishment item is, the more awful it ought to be for the human body.

Concerning the glycemic file rule, it separates nourishments into four fundamental classes regarding their capacity to raise the glucose. This capacity is presently estimated by the glycemic record GI that reaches from 0 to 100. (1) Foods that contain no carbohydrates and that have, in the outcome, an unimportant glycemic list (GI~0); people with diabetes may take them uninhibitedly. (2) Foods containing carbohydrates with a low glycemic index (GI 55 or less); individuals with diabetes ought to eat these items with some precautionary measures. (3) Foods that have carbohydrates of the high glycemic file (GI at least 56); people with diabetes must, so far as could be expected under the circumstances, reject them from their diet. (4) Processed nourishments; people with diabetes should counsel the producers' names to make sense of their specific glycemic list esteems.

Diabetics Top Best and Top Worst Foods

Expected for the individuals influenced by diabetes, the 'Diabetics Acid-Alkaline Food Chart' separates nourishments into six classifications. The rundown underneath goes from the top best to the topmost noticeably awful nourishments.

1. Alkalizing nourishment things with GI~0. They are among the top best nourishments. People with diabetes

may eat them uninhibitedly.

Asparagus; broccoli; parsley; celery; lettuce; carob; vegetable juices; mushrooms; squash; okra; zucchini; cauliflower; garlic/onions; green beans; beets; cabbage; crude spinach; lemons; avocados; limes; goat cheddar; herb teas; stevia; lemon water; ginger tea; green tea; canola oil; olive oil; flax-seed oil.

2. Alkalizing nourishment items that have a GI of 55 or less. Individuals who have diabetes should take them with balance, on account of their glycemic record.

Grain grass; sweet potato; carrots; crisp corn; olives; peas/soybeans; tomatoes; bananas; fruits; pears; oranges; peaches; grapefruit; mangoes; kiwi; papayas; berries; apples; almonds; Brazil nut; wild rice; chestnuts; coconut; quinoa; hazelnuts; lentils; soy milk; soy cheddar; goat milk; bosom milk; crude nectar; whey.

3. Acidifying nourishments with a GI~0. People with diabetes ought to expend them with an alert, being their acid-creating character.

Rhubarb; cooked spinach; pork; shellfish; liver; clams; meat; venison; sheep; cold-water fish; chicken; turkey; eggs; spread; buttermilk; curds; cheddar; corn oil; fat; margarine; sunflower oil; wine; lager; espresso; cocoa; tea; mayonnaise; molasses; mustard; vinegar; fake sugars.

4. Acidifying nourishments having a GI of 55 or less.

Considering both their acid-shaping element and their glycemic record, individuals with diabetes should eat them with limitations.

Lima beans; naval force beans; kidney beans; pinto beans; blueberries; cranberries; sharp fruits; prunes; plums; dark-colored rice; grew wheat bread; corn; oats/rye; entire wheat/rye bread; pasta/baked goods; wheat; pecans; peanuts; pistachios; cashews; walnuts; sunflower seeds; sesame; yogurt; cream; crude milk; custard; homogenized milk; dessert; chocolate.

5. Alkaline-framing nourishments with a GI of at least 56. As a result of their high glycemic file, these items are among the most exceedingly awful nourishments for people with diabetes. Along these lines, individuals who experience the ill effects of diabetes need to maintain a strategic distance from them.

Turnip; beetroot; tofu; potato with skins; figs; grapes/raisins; dates; melons; pineapple; watermelon; rice syrup; maple syrup; raw sugar; amaranth; millet.

6. Acid-creating nourishments with a GI of at least 56. These things are excessively acidic and have too high-glycemic list carbohydrates. They speak to the topmost noticeably awful nourishments for people with diabetes. In this way, people living with diabetes need to cut them totally from their dinners.

White bread; buckwheat; pumpkin; white rice;

spelled; potatoes w/o skins; white sugar; dark-colored sugar; prepared nectar; soda pops.

Acid-Alkaline Diet Benefits and Why It Is Recommended

On the off chance that you have known about the Atkins diet, at that point, the Acid Alkaline Diet is the direct inverse of that. The Atkins diet is a high protein, high fat, yet low carbohydrates diet. However, such foods tend to leave one low on energy, and they appear to be ill-advised gastronomically. An acid-alkaline diet then again isn't valuable for weight loss yet well beyond that is exceptionally gainful to the body working. An Acid alkaline, otherwise called an alkaline debris diet, alkaline acid diet, and the alkaline diet keeps the ph. The level of the body adjusted, thus defends against different ailments. Indeed, even ceaseless diseases like joint pain can be counteracted as well as restored if such a diet is pursued.

The premise of a diet that is acid-alkaline lies in the way that our body ph. in a perfect world ought to be a 7.3. This marginally alkaline degree of the body ph. Keeps all the essential organs working great, just as the assimilation of different minerals is improved at the point when this ph. Tilts to the acidic side difficulty begin blending. An acidic ph. Level prompts practically all body parts enduring in one manner or the other.

Presently since our body should be alkaline, it ought to reflect in our nourishment admission as well. Nourishments that are alkalizing ought to be devoured much more rather than the acidifying food sources.

Interpreted in a less complicated language, this would mean a higher amount of vegetable and organic product utilization and exceptionally low meats and oil consumption. On the off chance that the body's alkaline minerals, for example, calcium, magnesium, and potassium levels drop, so will its health making it ruffian and its safeguards to drop monitor. An alkaline diet shields that from occurring. An acid-alkaline or an alkaline debris diet involves 80% alkalizing nourishments and 20 % acidic nourishments. Since the acid-alkaline proportion in the body ought to be one is to four, our nourishment admission ought to be comparable.

An alkaline diet isn't just prescribed to shed those additional pounds but, at the same time, is and all the more significantly incredible methods for recapturing lost health and driving a more drawn out and more diseases free life. This diet is mainly prescribed to individuals who feel tired more often than not. Stress and a low energy level should both be possible away with acid-alkaline food. The individuals who experience the ill effects of constant viral fevers or the individuals who have a nasal clog more often than not can have healthier existences if they have an acid-alkaline diet.

Powerless nails, dryness, migraines, muscle torment, hives, joint torments, and a lot progressively such diseases discover their answer in an alkaline debris diet.

A more significant level of vegetable admission is suggested in an alkaline debris diet. Lemons ought to be pressed into water drinks. Millet or quinoa is favored over wheat, olive oil over vegetable oil and soups like miso are beneficial for following an alkaline debris diet. Lost health and force can be recovered, and numerous interminable sicknesses averted just as restored if an acid alkaline diet is pursued. It is a genuinely simple diet plan, which ought to adjust for a more drawn out and healthier life expectancy.

Alkaline Diet - What You Should Know About Its Health Benefits

The nourishment that we take today is very surprising from our precursors and is unique with what we are so acclimated with nowadays. How relevantly said, "We are what we eat." With the progression of innovation, the kinds of nourishments we expend made us dragged along. A view at the supermarket will stun you with passageways and paths of prepared nourishment things and creature items. With the simple accessibility of quick nourishments these days, there is no trouble in discovering one in our neighborhood.

Trend diets are by and large mostly to fault for presenting different dietary patterns; this incorporates high-protein diets. As of late, utilization of creature items and pure nourishment, things have expanded as an ever-increasing number of individuals forget about the everyday supply of foods grown from the ground in their diets.

It shocks no one why, nowadays, numerous individuals are experiencing various kinds of infirmities and hypersensitivities, for example, bone diseases, heart issues, and countless others. Some health specialists connect these diseases to the sort of nourishments we eat. There are specific sorts of nourishment that disturbs the equalization in our body that, during such occurrences, health issues emerge. On the off chance that no one but we could change our dietary patterns, it's far-fetched that aversion of diseases and reclamation of health can be accomplished.

Why Alkaline Is Important For Our Body

For a healthy body, the alkaline and acid apportion must be adjusted, which is estimated by the pH level in the body. PH esteems run from 0 to 14, and 7 is viewed as impartial. Any worth under seven is considered to be acidic. Pure nourishment, for example, meat and meat subsidiaries, pastries, and some improved drinks, as a rule, create an extraordinary measure of acid for the body. Acidosis, an instance of an elevated level of acidic in the circulation system and body cells, is the primary file for the ebb and flow various diseases dispensing numerous individuals. Some health experts reason that acidosis is liable for the underlying conditions endured by multiple people these days.

The alkaline or alkaline diet, which regularly presents in our body, kills the significant level of acidic in the body to accomplish harmony state. This is the primary capacity of the alkaline in the body. Be that as it may, the nearness of the alkaline in the body is immediately drained because of the elevated level of acidic substance it needs to kill, and there is deficient alkaline nourishment expended to renew the loss alkaline.

A Balance Alkaline-Acid Level For A Healthy Body

As portrayed beforehand, acidosis causes numerous health-related issues. A primary degree of acid gets into our framework, breaking the cells and organs when not kill appropriately. To forestall this, one must make sure that an equalization pH is kept up. To test whether our body contains a more significant level of alkaline can be completed quickly. This with the utilization of pH strips, which are realistic from any drug store. There are two kinds of pieces, one for the salivation and the other for a pee.

For the most part, a salivation pH level strip will decide the degree of acid your body is creating; the typical qualities ought to be somewhere in the range of 6.5 and 7.5 for the day. A pee pH level strip will show the degree of acid; a usual perusing ought to be somewhere in the range of 6.0 and 6.5 in the first part of the day and somewhere in the field of 6.5 and 7.0 around evening time.

Elevated Level of Acidity Is Harmful to the Body

On the off chance that you reliably experience the ill effects of weakness, cerebral pains, and having normal regular cold and influenza, these manifestations demonstrate an elevated level of acid in the body. The impact of acidosis in the body not just restrains the common diseases that we know yet different illnesses that you may endure is brought about by elevated levels of acid in the body.

Despondency, high acidity, ulcer, dry skin, skin break out, and overweight are a portion of those connected with the extraordinary degree of acidity in our body. Not restricted to these, other primary and genuine diseases, for example, joint diseases, osteoporosis, bronchitis, visit contaminations, and heart diseases. Indeed, even with meds, the manifestations might be masked and keep on influencing your health as the foundation of the issue has not been demolished. Taking more prescriptions will just exacerbate the problem as the mitigating drug will add to the acidic level in the body.

Alkaline Diet - A Sure Bet To A Healthy Body

To arrive at the base of the diseases, our frameworks' pH esteem must be kept up in a healthy state. Normally happening alkaline nourishments can enhance the lost alkaline levels in the body during the killing procedure. By keeping up a healthy alkaline diet, adequate measures of alkaline are recharged in the framework in this manner, taking the body back to the transcendent alkaline state.

So what are the approaches to incorporate an alkaline diet into our dietary patterns? The fundamental initial step is to diminish the measure of pure nourishment admission. As we know, these nourishments contain numerous synthetics, which are the guilty parties in expanding the acidic level in our body. The following stage is to eliminate the admission of meat and their subordinates and the measure of alcohol. The last advance is to build the rule of fresh foods grown from the ground, as they usually are high in alkalinity.

Oranges and lemons known for being acidic proselyte into alkaline after assimilation and consumed by the body is a decent alkaline diet. By and large, we should devour 75% of essential nutrients every day. The higher the measure of alkaline food we put into our framework, the more prominent the balance of the acidic condition in our body.

Why The Alkaline Diet And Cancer Is An Ideal Solution

Because of the scourge of cancer that has broken out as of late, there have been extraordinary steps made in where disease began, how it develops in the body, and how compelling an alkaline diet and cancer system has become. The meaning of cancer enables the patient to have some control in the counteractive action and skirmish of cancer cells. By adhering to an alkaline diet, this lessens and extinguishes, the creation of cancer and different diseases. Along these lines, an alkaline diet has been found to forestall illness, while an acidic food urges disease and cancer to develop.

At the point when you take the meaning of cancer just, it is 'a deformed cell.' This distorted cell can only imitate twisted cells, and since the human body recreates a vast number of cells day by day, the appropriate response is to stop that generation. The best resistance at that point is a decent offense, and that is the thing that an alkaline diet does as it encourages the high cells, while gagging out the disease.

The nourishments that are taken into the body ordinarily originate from two classifications - food sources that produce an acidic situation and food sources that provide an alkaline domain. On the off chance that you are taking a massive amount of drugs, this may make your framework lean more towards the acidic. However, it very well may be checked by devouring increasingly alkaline-creating nourishments.

An alkaline diet is commonly comprised of alkaline-delivering nourishments, with the goal that the pH level is brought to a degree of around 7.4. If you search online, there are alkaline/acidic graphs of the considerable number of nourishments. In the fact that you are merely starting this diet, duplicate the figure, and convey it with you when you shop or go out to eat. By and large, avoid handled nourishments, quick nourishments seared in trans-fat, any nourishment made with white sugar or white flour, and all nourishments with synthetic compounds and steroids. These nourishments all feed cancer cells. On the off chance that this is the thing that your diet is comprised of, check the basic nourishment rundown and see what to eat now.

Nourishments on that are alkaline-creating are vegetables, seeds, most natural products, dark-colored rice, and different grains, and fish. These nourishments can be blended and coordinated to your inclination for, at any rate, 80% of your perfect diet. Afterward, you include 20% of the acidic-creating food sources, and the acidic food sources are not all "terrible." Nourishments on the acidic side are entire grain loaves of bread, lean meats, milk and milk items, margarine, and eggs, and this signifies to make a 100% alkaline diet.

To screen your pH level once you have begun on an alkaline diet and cancer battling method for eating, check any health nourishment store for pH strips or litmus paper. There will be a shading diagram included to utilize and figure out what your pH blood level is. For a basic framework, it should enroll between 7.2 - 7.8. No two individuals are indistinguishable, so test your pH level about once every day as you begin. At that point, keep on checking once per week. On the off chance that you have to raise your pH level, eat increasingly alkaline nourishments, and utilize green enhancements. An alkaline diet will avert the disease usually.

Acid-Alkaline Diet - Will the Alkalizing Diet Help Fight Cancer and Other Diseases?

Alkaline is generally synonymous with its energy delivering properties, henceforth alkaline batteries. It is these equivalent energy-producing properties that have been incorporated into a diet rule. The alkalizing diet, additionally referred to in a few different names, for example, debris diet, acid alkaline diet, and the alkaline acid diet is a method of expending nourishment that will leave debris buildup consequently inciting a procedure like catabolized nourishments. Catabolize or catabolism put a way of separating atoms into basic waste in this manner, making energy.

While the diet sounds complex as a general rule, it isn't. Alkalizing foods rotate around basic guidelines, for example, expending a few new products of the citrus family, vegetables, vegetables, tubers, nuts, and low sugar-based organic products. Pretty much all the nourishment devoured and processed once discharged to the blood is either changed over into acids or alkaline. Individual cases to the alkalizing diet are organisms, sugar, caffeine, and liquor, just as a shirking of grains. The explanation for this particular case is that these nourishments, once processed, will transform into acid.

The objective of this diet is to help keep up the body's average pH level, which is around 7.35-7.45; this training guarantees steady alkalinity in the blood without focusing on the body's acid-base controllers. Not to say that the body can't keep up a pH level without this diet, while our framework will naturally do this for us, it is anyway kept up at a to some degree decent level that can effectively go from high to better or great to terrible. What makes the alkaline diet essential is that it gives the body an alternate wellspring of minerals like calcium from the bones rather than it plunging into these said stores.

As individuals age, the pH balance changes effectively. It can cause a decrease in renal capacities, and the alkaline diet keeps up the parity vital to stay away from this health decrease later on. Advocates of an alkalizing diet keep up that high acid creating nourishments can without much of a stretch upsets the fixed parity, consequently bringing about a loss in fundamental minerals, for example, magnesium, potassium, sodium, and calcium when the body attempts to reestablish its equalization.

Cerebral pains, nasal clog, laziness or absence of energy, uneasiness, peevishness, abundance mucous creation, anxiety, sores, steady colds or influenza are indications that alkalizing diet experts would consider trait as an individual with an imbalanced alkaline level. The diet isn't broadly polished at this point as most doctors don't accept that the decrease of acid-containing nourishment, for example, meats, salts, refined grains and dairies, and the expansion of an alkaline diet is entirely gainful for an individual's health.

Besides, specialists will likewise bring up that they are additionally questionable that acids in a person's diet are the primary driver of incessant ailments as guaranteed by alkaline diet devotees. It is anyway demonstrated that alkalizing foods do reduce the odds and help avert osteoporosis, muscle holding up realized by maturing, and the development of calcium stones in the kidney.

Approach to numerous individuals are confronting awful health issues, for example, cancer, diabetes, liver disease, hypertension, and that's just the beginning. Specialists over cure patients, and they become reliant on these meds. It is awful more individuals have not found out about the Alkaline Acid Diet. This diet encourages you to keep an alkaline body and equalization your bodies' pH. This diet is known to have cancer battling properties and enormous health benefits.

What Are the Benefits of Alkaline Diets?

Are you pondering about the advantages of alkaline diets? At that point, you're not the only one, because numerous individuals couldn't want anything more than to become familiar with this healthy method for eating. Yet, they simply aren't sure where to start learning the genuine article. That is the reason I'm giving you a manual to assist you with learning reality with regards to what alkaline diets are and the points of interest that you can appreciate.

This nourishment program is called a few distinct names, including the acid-alkaline diet, the alkaline diet, and the alkaline debris diet. These names all allude to similar essential ideas, which stress new vegetables, organic products, entire grains, vegetables, and healthy oils.

Why the Interest in Alkaline Diets?

Researchers understand that the breakdown of nourishments brings about results that can be either acid or alkaline, and that these side-effects can impact acid-alkaline parity in the body. The perfect pH of a healthy body is marginally alkaline, yet the more acid-delivering nourishments that are presented, the more acidic the body becomes. An acidic inside framework is in danger of various health issues.

An incredible, more significant part of the nourishments that the run of the mill individual eats today are profoundly handled, and they contain elevated levels of refined carbohydrates, unhealthy fats, sodium, and synthetic substances that add to health concerns. Sweet moves, meats, and cream cheddar all produce numerous acids when they are processed and assimilated. Prepared nourishments are another sort of item that expansion the nearness of acidic mixes. These acids are immediately discharged into the body's circulatory system, which makes issues as the body battles to keep up its regularly alkaline pH balance.

Specialists state that you ought to have a pH level in the scope of 7.35 to 7.45. Yet, with the exceptionally acidic American diet, it is hard to keep up a healthy pH level, as indicated by alkaline diet specialists. These defenders accept that by supporting the body with the sort of diet for which it was structured, better health and longer life can be accomplished. People are worked for a diet of crisp produce and other entire nourishments that have been exposed to negligible preparing.

What are the Benefits of Alkaline Diets?

As indicated by nourishment specialists, it is an acidic diet that is in any event somewhat liable for regular issues, for example, untimely maturing and constant sickness. Health conditions, for example, joint inflammation and kidney stones, are accepted to be connected to diets that are known to produce over the top measures of acids in the body.

Changing to a low-acid diet is accepted to be fit for expanding energy, diminishing bodily fluid, soothing side effects of fractiousness, and uneasiness. It may even prompt less cerebral pains and contaminations. Researchers are presently investigating cases that an alkaline diet can avoid bone loss, muscle squandering, urinary tract issues, and kidney stones.

Ask individuals who pursue these diets, and they'll disclose to you that they're healthier, more joyful, and more vivacious than their partners who seek all the more low-carb diets. A lot of individuals have discovered that their health issues have either diminished dramatically or been wiped out once they embraced alkaline foods. Shedding pounds is additionally a significant advantage for the individuals who consolidate entire nourishments into their ways of life.

Instructions to Get the Most Out of an Alkaline Diet

It tends to be useful to allude to a rundown of explicit nourishments, yet by and large, you should endeavor to eat a bounty of crisp foods grown from the ground each day. Plates of mixed greens are always a decent decision. Make a point to drink heaps of water, vegetable juice, or homegrown teas. Stay away from prepared nourishments, seared nourishments, chocolates, food sources that contain included sugars, and low-quality nourishments. Rather than adding sugar or salt to the nourishments you cook, have a go at utilizing healthy and delightful herbs and flavors. To wrap things up, remember that if you overcook your nourishments, you will lose a significant part of the dietary benefit.

Cancer Cells Does Not Live In An Alkaline Environment.

We are ever asked why the heart never gets cancer. The heart may get influenced in the end by cancer of some other piece of the body; however, we never know about cancer of the heart. This is because the heart never gets cancer. The alkaline diet is maybe the main perpetual approach to avoid and free oneself of cancer.

Let us comprehend what causes cancer and how an alkaline diet can counteract it. Every cell in our body takes in oxygen, supplements, and glucose while tosses out poisons. These cells are secured by a safe framework. Yet, as the body gets acidic, the invulnerable framework gets overwhelmed by the poisons, and the cell loses its ability to take in oxygen and, in this way, matures. This cell gets cancer influenced and is lost. The following inquiry is, would cancer be able to be forestalled and restored by devouring a diet with not so much acid but somewhat more alkaline. Cancer cells lie dormant in a ph of 7.4, yet as the body gets alkalized higher and the ph level arrives at 8.4, these threatening cells vanish. So the response to cancer lies in an incredibly alkaline diet. With the correct utilization prompting a high alkaline body ph, the cancer cells can't live in that condition and cease to exist.

Cancer cells being anaerobic can't live in oxygen. They can just flourish in low oxygen conditions. At the point when the ph of the body is kept up by expending an alkaline diet, the safe arrangement of the body remains solid. This prompts the cells getting enough oxygen and disposing of their poison squander. Cancer will neither flourish nor take birth under such conditions.

How does an alkaline diet avert cancer? Such a menu prompts a high alkaline body ph. This high alkaline body ph. brings about alkaline tissues in the body. Alkaline tissues hold multiple times more oxygen than acidic tissues. Cancer can't live in an oxygenated climate. On the off chance that the cells are oxygen-rich, they will avoid cancer. In this way, while an acidic tissue will be a perfect ground for cancer to create just as spread, an alkaline membrane will wreck a cancer cell. Having many green vegetables and organic products alongside alkaline water can spare you from cancer. To give your body, the best alkaline/acidic equalization expects one to eat nourishments that are profoundly alkalizing while at the same time staying away from the acidifying food sources.

An alkaline diet is extremely useful in battling numerous diseases separated from cancer. Alkaline enhancements are excellent approaches to remember alkaline nourishment for your diet. Overcooking of vegetables prompts their supplements being devastated. Alkaline improvements ensure one gets enough alkalizing nourishments in a day. Likewise, alkaline water is a decent option in contrast to conventional water. So on the off chance that you need your body to be sans cancer just as healthy and vivacious, receive an alkaline diet, and make it your lifestyle.

Health Benefits of an Alkaline Diet and Eating Alkaline Foods

An alkaline diet depends on standards of all-encompassing and Chinese medication, which have been utilized for quite a long time. An alkaline diet is roughly 75% alkaline nourishments and 25% acid food sources. On the off chance that the body is dangerous, it can take energy and cause weariness, have poor absorption, put on weight, have a throbbing painfulness, feel sick, and tired. An alkaline diet is a diet that underscores, to a changing degree, crisp organic product, vegetables, roots and tubers, nuts, and vegetables.

Grains, fish, meat, poultry, shellfish, cheddar, milk,

and salt all produce acid. These nourishments imply that the run of the mill Western diet is increasingly acid-creating. An alkaline diet is a questionable dietary convention dependent on the utilization of the crisp natural product, vegetables, roots and tubers, nuts, and vegetables and keeping away from grains, dairy, meat, and abundance salt, to adjust the acidity and alkalinity of one's body. Clinical examinations show that alkaline water is the ideal approach to acquire alkaline minerals, and acid waters like colas rapidly exhaust them. Our organs and organs work appropriately to the precise extent to the measure of alkaline and acid levels in our framework. Otto Warburg, a double-cross Nobel Prize victor, these acidic and harmful cells would then be able to get cancerous (he likewise expressed that these anaerobic cancer cells are crushed within sight of oxygen).

The most alkaline nourishments are products of the soil, and this is the reason a veggie lover and a natural diet is viable against numerous diseases. A vegan and natural diet not just accentuates nourishments that are alkaline, it likewise evades the most acid-delivering nourishments, creature proteins. This acid-alkaline equalization is significant because every real capacity, including breath, processing, and digestion, work best at specific pH levels. The general suggestion for lessening acidity by dietary methods incorporates keeping away from white bread, white sugar, pure oats, meat, fish, canned nourishments, tea, espresso, and toppings, while simultaneously expanding the utilization of products of the soil.

Citrus organic products alkalinity affect the body and ought to be devoured to help control acid reflux. One quart of alkaline water expended 45 minutes before eating supper is perfect for assisting in absorption and keeping away from acid reflux or indigestion. Apples, mangoes, bananas, citrus foods grown from the ground help keep up the body ph level at 7. Alkaline nourishments are raw low-sugar vegetables, lemons and limes, grew vegetables and vegetables, and developed seeds and nuts.

The American Journal of Clinical Nutrition presumed that alkalizing diets improve bone thickness and serum development hormone fixations; the acidosis coming about because of acidic foods adds to bone and muscle loss. The theory behind an alkaline diet is because our body's pH level is somewhat alkaline, with an ordinary scope of 7. The sustenance and good eating network have started to understand that what unique places into their body can affect how healthy they are by and large. Cerebral pains, headaches, tension, wretchedness, interminable weakness, asthma, stoutness, coronary illness, cancer, ADD, mental imbalance, and Alzheimer's everything conveys a shared factor: acid unevenness.

Alkaline Diet - How it Works

The alkaline diet is extremely the exact inverse of high fat, high protein, low carb diet that has become the standard as of late. On the off chance that you haven't known about an alkaline diet, you aren't the only one, yet it could profit you. On the off chance that you feel ineffective if you eat a diet low in carbs and high in protein, you ought to think about the alkaline diet. You ought to likewise consider on the off chance that you have manifestations of overabundance acidity. These indications incorporate interminable exhaustion, low energy, nasal blockage, visit contaminations or colds, apprehensive, on edge, focused on dry hair as well as skin, weak nails, muscle torment, leg issues, hives, and gastritis.

Before you start, you can gauge your salivary pH and see what it is. On the off chance that it's low, for example, a 4, at that point, this is an acidic outcome. If it's high, for example, an 8, at that point, this is alkaline. When you recognize what your pH is and you know which nourishments are alkaline and which are acidic, you can start to adjust things and return and keep up your body at alkaline ph. There are a few diagrams accessible online with the expectation of complimentary that can give the subtleties. How about we take a gander at barely any natural alkaline products - bananas, apples, coconut, nectarines, pineapple, and tomatoes are only a couple. Horse feed, celery, cabbage, carrots, garlic, lettuce, and mushrooms are a couple of alkaline vegetables. There are likewise alkaline dairy items, grains, and nuts.

How can it work? Most nourishments are either alkaline or acidic, relying upon the buildup they leave in the body and how they are processed. It's a smart thought to make progress toward an offset in the body with only slight alkalinity. You ought not to expect your diet is excessively acidic or too alkaline dependent on what you eat. Numerous things can influence the pH of the body. For instance, an orange is acidic when you feed it yet turns alkaline in the body. An alkaline diet that keeps the body marginally alkaline can profit you by improving your general health. There is a theory that it might prevent cancer cells from creating, and an alkaline diet has appeared to make some chemo drugs increasingly intense and progressively viable. It can assist you in recovering your health and stay disease-free. It can reestablish energy and essentialness and wipe out the nasal blockage, migraine, joint, and muscle torment.

Even though there may not be a lot of direct research on the alkaline diet, there is a lot of research that shows that individuals who are wiped out most occasions have acidic blood, which prompts a lopsidedness. Only sometimes is blood excessively alkaline, so you don't have to stress over eating such a large number of alkaline nourishments.

Here are a couple of test recipes.

Green Raw Soup

- 2 Avocados
- 1 Cucumber, strip, and seed
- 1 Jalapeno pepper, seeded
- 1 Yellow or red onion, diced
- Juice of 1/2 Lemon
- 1-2 cups Water or Veggie stock
- Two cloves broiled Garlic
- 1 Tbsp. Coriander
- 1 Tbsp. Parsley

Directions:

Puree all fixings (except onions) in a nourishment processor or blender. Add pretty much water to desired consistency. Top with diced onions for embellishing.

Pre-winter Tomato and Avocado Soup

Ingredients:

- Five large ready tomatoes.
- Two ready avocados
- 1/2 spring onion
- 1/4 cup ground almonds

- 1 cup juices from a characteristic vegetable stock without any additives or counterfeit added substances

- 1/4 teaspoon dill seed

- Run cayenne pepper

- Ocean salt and split dark pepper to taste.

Guidelines:

You should simply put the entirety of the fixings into a blender and mix! Spot the soup into a skillet and warm.

The alkaline diet may not be for everybody except is positively the correct decision for a few if you feel that the Alkaline diet could enable you to converse with your primary care physician before you start it.

Acid-Alkaline Diet - The Best Way to Balance Your Body

The acid-alkaline diet comes in various names. You may be confounded when you hear them. In any case, recall that they all relate to a specific something - knowing the nourishments that structure acid and those that structure alkaline side-effect. A portion of the well-known names is alkaline debris diet and alkaline acid diet. In light of the guideline of the arrangement, nourishments are characterized into three: acid, alkaline, or impartial. The response is controlled by knowing its answer with water.

Method of reasoning

Incidentally, when the prescription was not yet created, antiquated individuals satisfied 100 years of age. They live healthily in spite of the nonattendance of refined restorative types of gear and logical disclosures. Today, it is very occasional that you discover individuals who arrive at this age. You may feel this is something contrary to your desires, taking into account that science is further developed these days. If you attempt to look further, everything comes down to a certain something - diet.

Your diet is the essential motivation behind why you endure all the crippling diseases that are already obscure. Early individuals are eating, for the most part, products of the soil and almost no prepared nourishments. Yet, with the cutting edge innovation and quick-paced way of life, more individuals are including meat and handled items into their diet. These nourishment items are acid makers. As per the defenders of the acid-alkaline food, you should take nourishments that incorporate increasingly alkaline details rather than acid. This is because the blood is principally alkaline. It has a pH of 7.35 to 7.45. In light of their contentions, you need to keep up this normal pH to advance the most extreme health. This is because essential supplements are better caught up with a somewhat alkaline body liquid.

Advantages

An acid-alkaline diet gives a few health benefits. Besides the undeniable preferred position of keeping the pH parity of the body, it can assist rule with the trip a few diseases, including diabetes, cancer, and gastric issues. Different indications that can be precluded incorporate the accompanying:

- Loss of energy
- Nasal blockage
- Anxiety and apprehension
- Headache

What would be a good idea for you to do?

If you need to pursue the acid-alkaline diet, specialists guide you to take more leafy foods rather than meat, salt, and handled nourishments. These acid-delivering nourishments are the reasons why you experience the ill effects of various health issues.

Safety Concerns

Before you start with the acid-alkaline diet, you should initially counsel your primary care physician. Try not to take this sort of food on the off chance that you have kidney issues. This can just intensify your condition. You should likewise work intimately with your health care specialist on the off chance that you have previous health issues.

Instances of Alkaline-creating vegetables

- Barley grass, wheatgrass
- Beets, broccoli, cabbage, cauliflower
- Carrots, green peas, and beans
- Chlorella, lettuce, mushroom
- Celery, cucumber
- Eggplant, garlic, onion
- Pepper, pumpkin
- Spinach grows
- Sweet potato, tomatoes, watercress

Instances of acid-creating products of the soil

- Corn, lentils
- Olives, winter squash
- Legumes and beans
- Blueberries, cranberries
- Plums, Prunes
- Canned and coated organic products

Knowing the nourishments that acidify or alkalinize your blood will assist you in adjusting the inward pH of your body. Take the acid-alkaline diet today, and feel healthier and fitter.

Alkaline Diet Is Great

Just since the innovation of the pH scale, in 1909, have researchers had the option to quantify the acid level in the nourishment we eat. Even though before the change of the range, individuals knew there was increasingly acid in specific nourishments, they had no chance to get of knowing precisely how much. Researchers are present during the time spent better understanding alkaline nourishments and what it does to the body. The Alkaline diet depends on the menu of our predecessors, which had much increasingly natural plants and creature nourishment, as opposed to today when nearly everything is handled. Today, practically all the food we eat will give acid into the blood.

Nourishments, for example, grains, fish, shellfish, meat, poultry, cheddar, milk, and salt, are on the whole food sources that will cause the body to make acid. Since current society eats a ton of these nourishments, individuals' diets have been higher in acid. Since the blood has a pH level somewhere in the range of 7.35 and 7.45, the diet's theory is that the nourishment we eat ought to mirror this pH level too. Given this theory, individuals who pursue the alkaline diet will eat items to deliver the alkaline expected to get the pH level nearer to that of the blood.

Who is the Alkaline Diet For?

Due to the move in the populace to a diet higher in acid, individuals who have specific indications should attempt the alkaline diet to check whether it makes a difference. These manifestations include:

· Individuals who have no energy

· At the point when the body delivers an excess of bodily fluid

· Clogged nose

· Individuals who have incessant influenza and colds

· Individuals who are on edge, apprehensive and bad-tempered

· Individuals who have ovarian growths, polycystic ovaries, and amiable bosom sores

· Individuals who have incessant cerebral pains or headaches

What are alkaline diet nourishments?

Nourishments ordinarily proposed as alkaline diet nourishments are greens that contain a lot of supplements just as specific natural products, nuts, and different vegetables. The nourishments that usually are maintained a strategic distance from are grains, dairy, meat, sugar, liquor, caffeine, and organisms. Note that a portion of the nourishments on the rundown are high in acid before they are devoured; anyway, after the body digests it, they become a wellspring of alkaline.

Nourishments, for example, natural citrus products are acid; anyway, they have a great deal of alkalizing minerals. Crisp products of the soil are a case of nourishments that would be expended on the diet just as some entire grains, beans and vegetables, nuts and seeds, and healthy fats.

What are the Benefits of the Alkaline Diet?

Although the diet has the word diet before its name, it isn't really for individuals who need to get thinner; yet instead for individuals who wish to embrace a healthier way of life. The advantages of the alkaline diet are:

· Better processing

· Purifying the body normally

· The alleviation of joint inflammation and joint agony

· Gives the body more energy

· Enables an individual to get more fit

All that being stated, the alkaline diet returns us to the exit plan precursors ate, when the pH in their bodies was higher. This seems, by all accounts, to be a healthier method to eat, as it has been found to assuage numerous afflictions and has various advantages.

Acid-Alkaline Diet - The Top Seven Reasons to Go Alkaline and Avoid Acids

The body is a glorious device, and its bunch procedures and frameworks all interlock to make a streamlined machine that is intended to work with no glitches. Be that as it may, likewise, with all tools, the body needs the correct sort of fuel to work appropriately, and, when working appropriately, the waste items produced by consuming this fuel are flushed out with no issue.

Maybe once the body was splendidly adjusted, and perhaps humanity once lived in a flawlessly coordinated world, yet throughout the centuries, we have gotten lopsided; our diets and our biological system both turning out to be overpowered with acids and acidic squander. The issues related to over-acidification are numerous and differed, extending from weariness to joint pain to sadness and even cancer.

While there isn't a ton that should be possible about global contamination levels, in any event on an individual scale, we can control our diets and what we permit into our bodies. Holding fast to an alkaline diet may appear as though it requires a great deal of exertion and energy, yet the advantages of going - and remaining alkaline far exceeds the bothers. There are many motivations to start an alkaline diet, and it would take a book to show them all, yet the best seven motivations to go alkaline and keep away from acids have been recorded beneath.

1.) Weight Loss

This is a major one, for who hasn't had a weight issue at once or another? Furthermore, for the individuals who have, what might you have given for a straightforward, sheltered, and free approach to getting more fit?

The regular western diet and way of life are made out of such a large number of acid-creating substances (refined flours, sugars, meat, and dairy items) and propensities (smoking, liquor utilization, and physician endorsed drug use) that our bodies have gotten immersed with acid squanders. What's more, acids have an awful method for eating into and breaking down healthy muscle, tissues, and even organs.

One of the programmed guard instruments of the body is to deliver fat cells to shield our sensitive organs from these overabundance acids. The fat cells' capacity is to carry these acid squanders away from the organs and store it in less significant pieces of the body, however, as long as there are abundance acids in the body, the fat cells will stick to the organs protectively. When we can free ourselves of these abundance acids(through keeping up a high-alkaline diet, legitimate hydration, and exercise), the fat cells are never again required, and the body discharges them from obligation, bringing about weight loss.

2.) Increased Energy

The more acids that development inside the body, the

less the body's characteristic adjusting frameworks can process successfully, and the higher the body's acid levels become. What's more, the higher the acid levels become, the more alkaline minerals (calcium, magnesium, phosphates and so forth) will be filtered from the body's bones, muscles and tissues to verify that the blood can keep up the alkaline levels vital all together for the body to work. At the point when these sorts of alkaline minerals are expelled, effective digestion is repressed, bringing about drowsiness and weakness. The filtering of these sorts of minerals has likewise been connected to osteoporosis. When the acid levels are decreased through a legitimate diet and exercise, energy levels will increment.

3.) Alleviate Allergies

An acidic situation exhausts the safe framework and animates the invulnerable framework into what is known as "reaction mode." The final product of this being the body grows unimaginably increased affectability to a wide range of things; specks of dust, synthetic substances, and so on. This uplifted affectability we know as hypersensitivities. A portion of different ways that the body frees itself from over the top poisons, and acidic squanders is through irritation, expanding, skin inflammation, and abundance bodily fluid, everything that is identified with sensitivities. When the overabundance acids have been expelled from the body, the subtleties and their related manifestations will vanish.

4.) Reverse the Aging Process

Maturing is brought about by the development of acid squanders and the ensuing breakdown of substantial capacities. At the point when a body is too acidic, a condition called acidosis happens. Acidosis is, essentially, the over-worrying of oxidation frameworks and the breakdown of lipids. At the point when this happens, it discharges free radicals into the circulatory system. Free radicals are cells that assault cell dividers and films; executing the cell dividers and layers before at long last murdering the phones themselves. At the point when this happens, the apparent outcome is wrinkled, poor vision, age spots, awful memory, exhaustion, broken hormones; in short - untimely maturing. By expelling these acids, you can avert further harm to your cells and even invert the breakdown procedure.

5.) Oxidation

One of the symptoms of the development of acid squanders is that the body's cells don't get enough oxygen, and this causes a log jam in the entirety of the cell's heap of capacities. Much the same as the body itself, without enough oxygen, cells can kick the bucket. By dispensing with the acids that have been developed in your body by changing your diet and drinking alkaline water, you can re-start your blood.

6.) Decrease Blood Pressure

At the point when a body is excessively acidic, the cells start to hinder their capacities (see #5), and the heart needs to work all the harder to compensate for their drowsiness, this causes hypertension. Another reaction of high acidity in the development of plaque in the corridors and the diminishing of the width of the veins - which can likewise prompt hypertension. By expelling the acid waste develop from your framework, you can improve your cell working and take a portion of the weight off your heart.

7.) Decrease Chances of Developing Degenerative Diseases

To wrap things up, the development of acid squanders in the body (or Acidosis) is the underlying reason for practically all realized degenerative diseases including (yet not restricted to); diabetes, obesity, liver disease, kidney disease, cardiovascular disease, neurological diseases, untimely maturing, hormonal lopsided characteristics, osteoporosis and even most cancers.

Degenerative diseases flourish in acidic conditions, so by expelling their favored state, you can deny them of their capacity to duplicate or even to grab hold by any means.

What Can You Do?

On the off chance that you are genuinely keen on keeping up your health, or in switching any health issues you may have, there is one stage you can take at present, and that is to focus on an alkaline diet. By deciding to eat alkaline nourishments (new and crude vegetables, plates of mixed greens, natural alkaline products, seeds, nuts) and drinking alkaline water, you can free your body of years of gathered acidic burns through and turn around the hands of time.

Ideal Health Through the Alkaline Diet

The alkaline diet, acid alkaline diet, or alkaline acid diet is a kind of food that spotlights on the utilization of crisp vegetables, new organic products, root crops, tubers, vegetables, nuts, and every so often fish. By enjoying this sort of diet, it's accepted by the diet's specialists that we forestall the risks of acidity.

Returning To The Past

Ancient man expended a diet that bears little likenesses from the foods we devour today. Their diets comprised of wild vegetation and meat from prey. After the revelation of horticulture around 10,000 years prior, this diet changed.

After stone devices were created, grains turned into a reasonable nourishment source. When filtering and moving gadgets were designed, refined grains were presented. Dairy items were found when creatures were trained, thus did the measure of promptly accessible meat sources. Salt for enhancing was additionally found. During the mechanical upset, sugar as a sugar turned out to be mainstream.

The Reality

Nourishment, when processed, is either acidic or alkaline. There ought to be a harmony between the two. Sadly, because of the headways of horticulture and how we process nourishment and progress, we expend progressively acidic nourishment types contrasted with alkaline. The procedure that should keep us all around encouraged is, unfortunately, the reason for our very own end.

Blood coursing through our veins ought to be kept up somewhat alkaline. The pH levels in blood ought to in a perfect world be at 7.35 to 7.45. Professionals of the alkaline diet resolutely express that the type of food you eat will affect your general health. This implies acidic nourishment makes ready for diseases like diabetes and cancer, and alkaline framing nourishment makes available to consummate health.

Explanations behind Practicing Alkaline Diets

There are different reasons why individuals decide to go on an alkaline diet. Some go on a diet to get thinner. Some training the diet to overcome an ailment. Some training the diet to bring down the acidity levels in their body. Some do it for these reasons. Regardless, they decide to go on a diet to improve their health and prosperity.

Here are those reasons:

- Increase energy levels
- Prevention of bodily fluid generation
- Cure and avoidance of nasal blockage
- Cure and avoidance of ailments like flu
- Cure for peevishness and nervousness
- Cure and avoidance of interminable cerebral pains
- Prevention of the backslide of genuine diseases like cancer

Genuine, the therapeutic world neglects to approve the viability of the diet. Be that as it may, one reality remains. The acid shaping western diets is the primary driver of certain diseases like obesity, diabetes, and cancer. Hence, we can securely derive that the alkaline diet is the best approach to consummate health.

Why the Alkaline Diet Beats Low Carb

The alkaline diet is a method for eating that spotlights on nourishments that move your interior pH toward the soluble finish of the range. This theory isn't new, yet its ubiquity has dramatically expanded over the previous decade, and intrigue keeps on developing. Many are bewildered because the words "alkaline" and "alkalizing" are two distinct things. This is to state that nourishment that preferences extremely acidic, for example, lemon juice or apple juice vinegar, can have an unequivocally alkalizing impact once it has been processed and absorbed. By a similar token, nourishment that preferences sweet instead of acidic, for example, pure sweetener, is regularly unequivocally acidifying once it has been ingested.

The Alkaline Diet versus Well known Low-Carb Diets

If you have considered difficult the alkaline diet, you might be thinking about how it appears differently about other healthy diets, especially low-carb diets, including the Atkins diet and the South Beach diet.

At first, the alkaline diet is by all accounts the perfect inverse of the low-carb diet, however actually progressively mind-boggling. As you are continually reminded, the low-carb diet confines your admission of carbs, including bread, pasta, potatoes, sugar, beans- - even foods are grown from the ground. Then again, you are permitted to eat as much as you need with regards to pork skins, cheddar, and different nourishments that are wealthy in protein and fat.

Conversely, the alkaline diet confines the utilization of meat and dairy items, about all nourishments that make the body increasingly acidic. Another distinction is that while low-carb diets limit products of the soil, these nourishments are unequivocally energized on the alkaline diet. This is because the new product has the most supplements and the least calories of any nourishment, making it an unquestionable requirement have for any individual who needs to support energy and get in shape.

Shockingly, in any case, alkaline and low-carb diets do share something. The two foods urge individuals to eat less sugar and handled grains, yet for various reasons. Enthusiasts of the low-carb diet call attention to that these bottomless carbs are a significant explanation that individuals have gotten such a considerable amount of fatter in recent decades. In the expressions of diet master Barry Sears, the focal walkways of any supermarket are fundamentally one major piece of carbs split into various packs and boxes. (There's a ton of fat in those bundles, as well.)

Strikingly, these handled carbs additionally will, in general, be acidifying. This is because the most well-known grains, to be specific corn, rice, and wheat, contain acidifying mixes.

At the point when you get down to it, the primary contrast between these two diets is that the low-carb diet takes a heavy hammer to carbs, while the alkaline diet utilizes a surgical tool. Genuine, some carbs are destructive, especially when you eat a lot of them. Yet, something isn't right when against carb delirium arrives at such a pitch, that individuals evacuate even apples, carrots, and celery from their diets. These nutritious nourishments are profoundly gainful, and they're certainly not why such a large number of individuals are fat. Despite what might be expected, they are the way to getting more fit since they top you off without adding numerous calories to your day by day consumption.

CHAPTER THREE
THE ALKALINE DIET METHOD AND WEIGHT LOSS

Dr. Sebi Diet Weight Loss

This part is clear as crystal. Weight loss will undoubtedly happen when following the diet because the Dr. Sebi diet comprises of common vegetables, organic products, grains, nuts, and vegetables. It disposes of waste, dairy, meat, and handled nourishment, so usually, you will shed pounds. The Dr. Sebi diet fills in as a cleanser and receives numerous rewards, including your body expressing gratitude toward you.

Solid Immune System

A powerless invulnerable framework is the consequence of ailments and diseases. Some cases that they have fortified their insusceptible framework and have been mended of specific sicknesses by following the Dr. Sebi diet reliably, and we, as a whole, realize that medication doesn't fix diseases.

Diminished Risk of Disease

Acidic nourishments dissolve the mucous film of the cells and internal dividers of the body, which prompts an undermined framework that makes disease conceivable and a fix inconceivable. Accordingly, eating alkaline nourishments can diminish the danger of illness and help your body in getting what it needs to encourage high cells.

Lower Risk of Stroke and Hypertension

As indicated by the National Institute of Health (NIH), first-line treatments for all phases of hypertension incorporate exercise and weight loss. In any case, results from one microscopic cross-sectional examination propose that a plant-based diet is a more significant intercession than medication and standard therapeutic practice. Regular Health has additionally talked about the advantages of a plant-based diet in contrast with medicine, expressing that a plant-based diet can diminish plaque in the veins and lower danger of diabetes, stroke, and coronary illness in restorative research they have investigated.

Energy

Diets overwhelming in meat, dairy, and white sugar can be a drag on your body and energy levels. Concentrating on plant-based living is a superior approach and can upgrade the energy that you show all the time.

Expanded Focus

Following Dr. Sebi's lessons will clear cerebrum

haze, keep you engaged, and less annoyed by upsetting circumstances that emerge. Regardless of whether you are not wiped out, utilizing a plant-based methodology will assist you with carrying on with a long and healthy life.

Test menu

Here is a three-day test menu on the Dr. Sebi diet.

Day 1

• Breakfast: 2 banana-spelled hotcakes with agave syrup

• Snack: 1 cup (240 ml) of green juice smoothie made with cucumbers, kale, apples, and ginger

• Lunch: kale plate of mixed greens with tomatoes, onions, avocado, dandelion greens, and chickpeas with olive oil and basil dressing

• Snack: natural tea with organic product

Supper: vegetable and wild-rice pan sear

Day 2

• Breakfast: shake made with water, hemp seeds, bananas, and strawberries

• Snack: blueberry biscuits made with blueberries, unadulterated coconut milk, agave syrup, ocean salt, oil, and teff and spelled flour

• Lunch: natively constructed pizza utilizing a spelled-flour outside, Brazil-nut cheddar, and your selection of vegetables

- Snack: tahini margarine on rye bread with cut red peppers as an afterthought
- Dinner: chickpea burger with tomato, onion, and kale on spelled-flour flatbread

Day 3

- Breakfast: cooked quinoa with agave syrup, peaches, and unadulterated coconut milk
- Snack: chamomile tea, seeded grapes, and sesame seeds
- Lunch: a spelled-pasta serving of mixed greens with hacked vegetables and olive oil and critical lime dressing
- Snack: a smoothie made with mango, banana, and unadulterated coconut milk
- Dinner: generous vegetable soup utilizing mushrooms, red peppers, zucchini, onions, kale, flavors, water, and powdered kelp

This example feast plan centers around the endorsed fixings remembered for the diet's healthful guide. Suppers on this arrangement accentuate vegetables and natural products with modest quantities of the other nutrition classes.

The Dr. Sebi diet advances eating entire, natural, plant-based nourishment. It might help weight loss on the off chance that you don't typically eat like this. Nonetheless, it intensely depends on taking the maker's costly enhancements, is exceptionally prohibitive, does not have certain supplements, and mistakenly vows to change your body to an alkaline state. In case you're hoping to pursue a more plant-based eating design, numerous healthy diets are progressively adaptable and practical.

The Alkaline Diet: A Little-Known and Powerful Weight Loss Plan

Imagine a scenario in which you thought about a weight loss program that would assist you with getting in shape and feel more youthful. OK, attempt it? The alkaline diet and way of life have been around for more than 60 years, yet numerous individuals aren't acquainted with its regular, protected, and demonstrated weight loss properties!

The alkaline diet isn't a contrivance or a prevailing fashion. It's a healthy and straightforward approach to appreciate new degrees of health. In this post, you'll find out about what this dietary arrangement is, the thing that makes it unique, and how it can create groundbreaking outcomes for you, your waistline, and your health. It is right to say that you are getting a charge out of a thin and attractive body today? Assuming this is the case, you're in the minority.

Unfortunately, more than 65 percent of Americans

are either overweight or hefty. In case you're overweight, you presumably experience indications of ill health like weakness, expanding, sore joints, and a large group of different signs of unexpected frailty. More terrible yet, you most likely want to abandon regularly getting a charge out of the body you need and merit. Maybe you've been informed that you're merely getting more established, yet that necessarily isn't reality. Try not to get tied up with that falsehood. Different societies have healthy, lean seniors who appreciate excellent health into their nineties!

Indeed, your body is a splendidly planned machine, and on the off chance that you have any side effects of ill health, this is a sure sign that your body's science is excessively acidic. Your side effects are only a weep for help. This is because the body doesn't merely separate one day. Slightly, your health disintegrates gradually after some time, at last falling into 'dis-ease.'

What's going on with how you're eating now?

The Standard American Diet (S.A.D.) centers around refined carbohydrates, sugars, liquor, meats, and dairy. These nourishments are largely exceptionally acid-shaping. In the interim, in spite of supplications from the nourishing specialists, we just don't eat enough of the alkalizing nourishments, for example, crisp organic products, veggies, nuts, and vegetables. To put it plainly, our S.A.D. way of life disturbs the universal acid-alkaline parity our bodies need. This condition causes stoutness, low-level a throbbing painfulness, colds and influenza, and inevitably disease sets in. We've lost our direction. This is the place an alkaline diet can help reestablish our health.

• I'm sure you're acquainted with the term pH, which alludes to the degree of acidity or alkalinity contained in something. Alkalinity is estimated on a scale. You can take a necessary and reasonable test at home to see where your alkalinity level falls, just as to screen it routinely.

• Medical analysts and researchers have known for in any event 70 years this lesser-known fact. Your body requires a specific pH level, or sensitive parity of your body's acid-alkaline levels - for ideal health and imperativeness.

You may think..."I don't have to know this science. Besides, what does the best possible pH parity and alkalinity matter to me?" I know these were my inquiries when I initially found out about alkaline eating.

We'll utilize two instances of how acid and alkalinity assumes a job in your body.

1. We, as a whole, realize that our stomach has acid in it. Alongside proteins, this acid is fundamental for breaking nourishment into essential components that can be consumed by the stomach related tract. Consider the possibility that we didn't have any acid in our stomachs.

We would kick the bucket from lack of healthy sustenance right away because the body couldn't use an entire bit of meat or a whole bit of anything, so far as that is concerned! Bode well?

2: Different pieces of our body require various degrees of acidity or alkalinity. For instance, your blood requires a somewhat more alkaline level than your stomach acids. Consider the possibility that your blood was excessively acidic. It would eat through your veins and conduits, causing a substantial inward drain!

While these models exhibit that the different parts or frameworks in the body need distinctive pH levels, we don't have to stress over that.

Our concern is primary, and it's this. We are essential to acidic, generally speaking, period. In case you're keen on getting familiar with pH, you can discover massive amounts of data on the web by basically looking through the term.

The most significant thing to know is this. At the point when your body is too acidic over quite a while, it prompts numerous diseases like stoutness, joint pain, bone thickness loss, hypertension, coronary illness, and stroke. The rundown is unending because the body essentially surrenders the fight for imperativeness and goes into endurance mode as long as it can.

An alkaline diet is unique.

Numerous diets center on similar nourishments that cause you to be overweight or debilitated in any case. They solicit you to eat less from those things, to eat additional time every day, or to join them quickly.

Indecency to these diet's makers, they realize that vast numbers of us would prefer not to roll out the more significant improvements for our health. We like food that is centered on prepared and refined nourishments, our meat, our sugar, alcohol, and such. The diet makers are attempting to assist us with rolling out more uncomplicated improvements.

We've become acclimated to eating along these lines, and it's not ALL our deficiency! Insatiable nourishment preparing monsters have a personal stake in keeping us eating along these lines. Benefits are a lot higher in this area of the nourishment business than in the generation of your progressively fundamental nourishments like foods grown from the ground.

In this way, once more, YES...this diet is extraordinary. On the off chance that those different diets worked, you would feel lean, healthy, and crucial. You wouldn't have to peruse this article. You wouldn't require a dietary change.

Here's a fractional rundown of nourishments that you can eat unreservedly in an alkaline diet:

• Fresh foods grown from the ground made juices

- Fresh veggies and juices
- Cooked veggies
- Some vegetables and soy
- Lean proteins and a few eggs
- Certain grains
- Healthy fats and nuts

*You might be astonished to discover that a few veggies and organic products are preferred for you over others!

You can expend constrained amounts of these nourishments and refreshments:

- Dairy
- Many normal grains
- Refined nourishments and sugars
- Alcohol and caffeine

What's it like to be on the alkaline diet, and what results would you be able to anticipate?

Like any adjustment in diet or way of life, you'll experience a modification period, however, because you're consuming the cleanest fuel, which your body pines for, so not at all like many diet plans, you won't ever need to feel hungry. Also, you can eat all you like until you're fulfilled. You likewise won't have to check calories. What's more, you'll appreciate a lot of assortment, so you'll never get exhausted with eating.

Think about an alkaline diet as a sort of 'juice quick' for the body. Just it's not all that outrageous. You're eating supplement thick, effectively absorbable nourishment that your body wants. When you give every one of the cells of the body that it so frantically needs, your craving leaves. Also, there's no compelling reason to stress over exhausting veggies since there are vast amounts of delightful recipes found on the web and in books.

With all the diet designs out there, for what reason would it be advisable for you to consider an elective arrangement like the alkaline diet?

When pursued appropriately, you can hope to liquefy the fat away more effectively than with conventional plans. Numerous tributes exist where individuals report shedding more than two pounds every week. (Furthermore, that much weight wouldn't be intelligent in most diet programs.) Plus, your skin will turn out to be increasingly supple once more, your energy will increment, and you'll feel more youthful.

Furthermore, the alkaline diet does two significant things that conventional diets don't.

1. It gives better sustenance than your body's cells.

2. It detoxifies typically and cleanses the cells, as well.

These two certainties are behind the motivation behind why an alkaline diet works so rapidly and securely.

One last note, while thinking about an alkaline diet. Since it tends to's be unique about how you might be accustomed to eating, you may think about whether you can come back to your previous dietary patterns. The legit answer is that it's keen to proceed with the same number of the standards as you can once you have lost all your weight. Be that as it may, it shouldn't be win big or bust. Anything you do to receive a healthier diet will significantly expand your odds of keeping the weight off for good. I'm a significant defender of eating an alkaline diet more often than not. I'm enthusiastic about it since it worked for me, and helped turn my weight and my health around. When you pursue an alkaline diet for a month or two, you can decide the amount of it you need to embrace as a significant aspect of your long haul healthy way of life.

Acid to Alkaline Diet, How to Lose Weight and Live a Healthier Lifestyle Naturally

Acid to Alkaline Diet

The acid to alkaline diet is turning into a more discussed subject these days, yet at the same time, most of the populace are unconscious of what it is. Individuals who bite the dust youthful, have health issues, experience the ill effects of heftiness and so on., by and large, have an extremely acidic inside condition though individuals who live to mature age and don't experience the ill effects of genuine health issues have an interior situation that is increasingly alkaline.

In the cutting edge Western world by far, most of the individuals carry on with an unhealthy way of life, overwhelmingly eating garbage and unhealthy nourishment and being always presented to different variables that drastically negatively sway our health, in drastic differentiation to the acid to an alkaline diet. As per the World Health Organization (WHO), there are more than one billion overweight grown-ups around the world, with around 300 million of them clinically fat. This measurement is unnerving and is dramatically expanding ordinary!

As a health care expert myself, individuals regularly ask me what the ideal approaches to remain healthy are. I usually tell my patients that with the goal for us to carry on with a healthy life, not be overweight, maintain a strategic distance from a specific disease and sicknesses and by and large live to a past age with essentialness and force, it is fundamental that we focus on the acid to an alkaline diet. By watching your bodies pH levels and eating in like manner to guarantee your body is more alkaline than acidic, individuals experience things like fast weight loss (by a quickened fat transfer process), they will live more, feel less pushed, have an improved insusceptible framework, show signs of improvement and increasingly relaxing rest, have more energy and can likewise encounter an expansion in charisma. These advantages alone are critical to health, life span, and happy life. By enabling the body to detox like this through the acid to an alkaline diet, individuals additionally have an expanded capacity to retain nutrients and minerals and help dodge numerous frightful diseases, including cancer and joint inflammation. With a progressively alkaline body, stress, and weight on the inward organs is facilitated, skin, bones, and cells recover and help keep you young.

Then again, if an individual's body is too acidic they can without much of a stretch encounter weight by picking up and clutching fat, they will age snappier, an absence of energy will be healthy, they will effectively and reliably draw in disease and infection's and make an inside situation where yeast and microorganisms can undoubtedly flourish.

Most of the individuals living in the Western world don't pursue an acid to an alkaline diet and are commonly more on the acidic scale. This is generally expected in our menu. Eating things like shoddy nourishment, burgers, bubbly drinks, having a high sugar consumption, singed food sources, unnatural organic product juices, impersonation nourishments, energy drinks, and prepared food sources, for instance, all push our bodies inside condition down on the acidic scale. There are even some generally healthy nourishments to know about, strawberries, mangos, and peaches, for instance, are high in sugar, in this manner make an acidic situation in the body. Some different astonishments that likewise cause acidic to develop incorporate rice, fish, oats, and cheddar, so these nourishments are to be constrained when following an acid to an alkaline diet. This is one motivation behind why it is essential to know what nourishments will cause an acid response and which will make you increasingly salty. Different contemplations that likewise cause our bodies to be increasingly acidic incorporate various synthetics, tobacco, radiation, pesticides, fake sugars, air contamination, liquor, drugs, and stress.

Ideal pH to get every one of the advantages of alkalinity is 7.4pH. If your body goes, 3-4 focuses whichever way you will pass on! The pH scale is as per the following:

0 = complete acid/sulfuric acid, hydrochloric acid

1 = gastric juices

2 = vinegar

3 = lager

4 = wine, tomato juice

5 = downpour

6 = milk

7 = unadulterated water

8 = ocean water

9 = preparing pop

10 = cleanser, milk of magnesia

11 = alkali, lime water

12 = dye

13 = lye

14 = Total Alkaline/Sodium Hydroxide

The acid to the alkaline diet will enable your body to remain at the ideal range, around 7.4pH. The body's response to attempting to keep this acid, alkaline parity, is both fantastic and exciting. At the point when your body is too acidic, it has a go at everything to get to an increasingly alkaline state. At the position when this happens, the body stores some acid in your fat to prevent it from doing damage to our body, which is something to be thankful for, yet your body at that point clutches the fat for security, making the individual put on weight. When there is abundance acid inside, the body finds alkaline somewhere else from your bones and teeth, yet your bones and teeth get so drained that they become delicate and begin to rot. This can prompt numerous diseases of the bones and teeth, including joint inflammation and tooth rot. This would not occur if an individual were following an acid to an alkaline diet.

The development of acid, for the most part, will settle away from your healthier organs; however, instead, it floats towards your weakest organs that are as of now inclined to disease. It resembles a pack of wolves searching for the lowest among the group, taking out the simple prey. As your flimsier organs are focused on, it makes it a lot simpler for certain diseases to set in, including cancer. Realize that cancer cells become lethargic on the off chance that you are at 7.4pH (which is the body's ideal pH levels), therefore further underlining the significance of keeping up a healthy pH level in our bodies by following the acid to an alkaline diet. When there is acid in the framework, it additionally taints your circulatory system. This like this forestalls the types of blood capacity to deliver oxygen to the tissues. RBC's are encompassed by a negative charge so they can skip off one another and move around in the blood rapidly and give their decency.

However, when you are too acidic, they lose their negative charge, and they remain together, making them move gradually. This makes them battle to deliver supplements and oxygen in our framework. One of the primary manifestations of this harming is you begin to feel a loss of energy even though you are getting enough rest. Beginning an acid to the alkaline diet can address this rapidly. Your blood likewise has this response in the wake of drinking liquor. We should place this into point of view; it takes around 33 glasses of water to kill one glass of coke! I'm not, in any case, going to refer to the stuff to destroy a portion of different things that we are placing into our bodies, I think you get the image!

One incredible approach to reliably make your body progressively alkaline is by having green drinks each day. They are straightforward to make, taste extraordinary and are pressed with nutrients, minerals, and chlorophyll, which fuel our body. Chlorophyll is a significant piece of the acid to an alkaline diet and is the green blood of plants. It is a fantastic detoxify-er, blood manufacturer, cleaner, and oxygen promoter. Indeed, the advantages of chlorophyll on our bodies are very various to remember for this article. There are numerous recipes for making delicious green drinks. The one I am right now having regular is as per the following; 2 apples, four sticks celery, 1/3 cucumber, a large bunch of child spinach leaves, and one avocado. I have been doing this ordinary (pretty much) for about the most recent a half year, and not once have I been wiped out. I have additionally seen an expansion in energy, and I am likewise profiting by increasingly peaceful rest. On the off chance that you genuinely need to shed pounds that stay off for good, help your energy, and improve the general nature of your health and your life, then you should look at the acid to an alkaline diet, as it is essential to accomplishing that.

Utilizing an Alkaline Diet for Weight Loss

Numerous individuals endeavor prevailing fashion diets or those which guarantee snappy outcomes trying to get in shape. These diets may create brings about the present moment, yet after some time, this can be an exceptionally unhealthy approach to get thinner. Also, numerous individuals recover the weight when they go off their exacting diet. At the point when an acid diet is utilized for weight loss and control, it is all the more a way of life change. The outcomes may not occur without any forethought. However, the weight won't be recovered. An alkaline diet is wealthy in nourishments, which are generally low in calories, for example, most vegetables and natural products. A significant number of the nourishments that are high in fat and calories are likewise acidifying, so when these nourishments are expelled from the diet, a characteristic and healthy weight loss will happen. These nourishments incorporate red meat, greasy food sources, and high-fat dairy items, for example, whole milk and cheddar, sugar, pop, and liquor. When you quit eating these nourishments, your body will be a lot healthier, less acid, and you'll additionally get more fit all the while. Since the diet is healthy, you can stay with it long haul. Numerous individuals who start an alkaline diet exclusively to get in shape find countless different advantages. An expanded energy level, protection from an ailment, and a general improvement in health and prosperity are among the numerous benefits you can understand on an alkaline diet.

The most effective method to Start an Alkaline

Diet

Numerous individuals find that it is simpler to begin an alkaline diet by rolling out little improvements. Start by gradually decreasing the measure of meat, sugar, and fat in your diet, while including crisp organic products, vegetables, healthy fats, for example, olive oil, almonds, soy items, and normal sugars, for instance, Stevia. You'll discover after some time, your preferences will change, and you'll begin to lean toward this sort of diet.

Would you be able to Use an Alkaline Diet For Weight Loss?

How Your Body Handles Acid

Anyway, for what reason would anyone care about being on an alkaline diet in any case? Well, the explanation is necessary. As a populace, we are tossing our bodies out of equalization by ingesting poisons, for example, pop and creature proteins in mass amounts. Subsequently, acid is developed in such enormous quantities that the body goes into endurance mode. While acid would ordinarily be handled and expelled by the liver and kidneys, when a lot of it exists, the body stores it in fat to save the health of your organs. The outcome is an unequal measure of acid and dehydration in the body. The body's homeostasis exists at a pH estimation of 7.3. Standard (unbiased) water has a pH of 7.0. The capacity to ionizer water and devour an alkaline diet has incredible advantages for your health.

However, for what reason is an alkaline extraordinary for weight loss? A horde of advantages has been ascribed to keeping up your body's normal ph. Turning around the impacts of continuous diseases, for example, diabetes, acid reflux, angina, headaches, and joint inflammation, are a couple of the significant advantages. Liberating people with diabetes from their insulin crazed appetite fits has brought about a lot of weight loss. However, you'll see that even typical individuals have seen incredible weight loss because of an alkaline diet. At the point when the body is liberated of its harmful express, your digestion can work all the more productively. Fat and proteins are scorched and put away appropriately. Likewise, individuals have seen the advantages of expanded energy and sex drive, enabling them to be increasingly dynamic and gainful.

Improving Your Alkaline Diet for Weight Loss

If you are endeavoring to utilize an alkaline diet for weight loss, it is significant you realize how to adopt the fair strategy. In the fact that you use alkaline water and alkaline nourishments related to a healthy way of life, you will get the "wonder" weight loss that everybody is raving about. When you start drinking the alkaline water all the time, you can move from drinking water with pH 9.0 to pH 9.5 (for grown-ups). Expending a good measure of this high pH water is ensured to help the body in coming back to acid-alkaline congruity.

Additionally, you should utilize the high pH water while getting ready nourishments like soup and stews, to adjust the acidifying creature proteins or other acidic parts of the nourishment.

In the above, you have perceived how you can utilize an alkaline diet for weight loss, yet there is significantly more to be scholarly. To guarantee that you are going to lose weight, it is significant you find out about alkaline nourishments. The absolute most acid-filled nourishments would be the ones you wouldn't dare hoping anymore. Numerous dairy items, for instance, are exceptionally high in acid substance.

Alkaline Diet for Health and Weight Loss

There are a ton of insane diets available that guarantee to assist you with shedding pounds. Shockingly, on the off chance that you take a gander at the healthy benefit of a portion of these diets, they are regularly seriously deficient. If you have to get thinner, you ought to do it while eating food that is useful for your body, with the goal that you will get healthier rather than merely more slender. An alkaline diet is a healthy way to deal with weight loss that will keep you stimulated, healthy, and inspired to drop the pounds.

An alkaline diet is not the same as different diets since it centers mostly around the impact that nourishments have on the acidity or the alkalinity of the body. At the point when nourishments are processed and used by the body, they produce what is usually alluded to as an "alkaline debris" or "acid debris." The first pH of the nourishment doesn't factor into this decisive impact inside the body. The absolute most acidic nourishments, for example, organic citrus products, really produce an alkaline effect when eaten. At the point when increasingly alkaline nourishments are eaten instead of acid nourishments, the pH of the body can be acclimated to an ideal degree of roughly 7.3. While this isn't incredibly alkaline, it is sufficient to receive numerous healthful rewards.

Alkaline Diet - How Does It Help?

The alkaline diet, otherwise called Alkaline Acid Diet, is diet-dependent on the utilization of nourishment. For example, natural products, vegetables, roots, nuts, and vegetables, however, maintain a strategic distance from dairy, meat, grains, and salts. As of late, this diet has picked up fame among diet and nourishment experts and creators. It is still in banter on the productivity of the alkaline diet because there is no solid proof that the alkaline diet can decrease certain diseases.

As previously mentioned, organic products, vegetables, roots, nuts, and vegetables are a piece of an alkaline diet. This is because this nourishment discharged alkaline in the wake of being processed, assimilated, and used. Then again, dairy, meat, grains, and salts produce acid after the procedures. Nourishment is classified as acid-delivering or alkaline-creating dependent on their pH (intensity of Hydrogen) values, where pH 0 - 6 is acidic, pH 8 - 14 is alkaline, and pH 7 is nonpartisan (water). Consequently, the alkaline diet alludes to the menu of having a more significant amount of alkaline-delivering nourishment.

Alkaline Diet

Our blood has a pH somewhere in the range of 7.35 and 7.45, which is marginally alkaline. Alkaline diet depends on this pH level of our blood, and any food that is high in acid-delivering nourishment will disorganize the equalization. At the point when the body attempts to rejuvenate the harmony of pH in the blood, the acidity of the food will add to the loss of crucial minerals, for example, potassium, magnesium, calcium, and sodium. The irregularity will make individuals vulnerable to sickness.

Sadly, Western diets are progressively acid-delivering, and they expend minimal new foods grown from the ground. Because of the approach of the alkaline diet, the standard of the Western diet has changed impressively. Some diet and nourishment professionals accept that acid-delivering diet may cause some constant ailment and following manifestations, for example,

· Migraine

· Lazy

· Visit influenza and cold, and overabundance mucous generation

· Tension, apprehension

· Polycystic ovaries, ovarian sores, considerate bosom growths

Albeit some accept the above conditions are the consequence of acid-delivering diet and utilization of products of the soil is valuable to health, a few specialists believe that acid-creating diet doesn't cause persistent disease. Other than that, there are proofs demonstrated that alkaline foods forestall the development of calcium kidney stones, osteoporosis, and age-related muscle squandering.

Equalization diet

Albeit an alkaline diet is liked, it isn't prescribed to have an extreme diet (eat all alkaline-delivering nourishment). It is healthier to take a stab at a reasonable center ground of the two kinds of food. Simply make sure to observe the pointers above and counsel a specialist/specialist before you need to attempt another diet.

Step by step instructions to Lose Weight With an Alkaline Diet and Alkaline Foods

Those battling with abundance weight see many

commercials of thousands of weight loss items. However, a large portion of these individuals never knows WHY they are overweight in any case. Numerous individuals like to have more energy for the day, yet the tidbits and stimulated drinks that many expend are exceptionally acid-shaping.

What Excess Acidity Does Inside The Body

By making acidity in blood, tissue, and body cells, these ordinary tidbits (just as cheap food, handled nourishment, desserts, all yeast containing items, and so forth.) may meddle with healthy energy creation and frequently bring about ensuing weight gain. The purpose behind that is the body's reaction to overabundance acidity: it stores acid squanders in fat cells to keep them from essential organs.

The over-acidification/acidosis of our body cells is the purpose behind numerous diseases, will hinder cell exercises and works, and is the thing that prompts overweight: to shield itself from conceivably genuine harm, the body makes new fat cells to store the additional acid. Be that as it may, when the acidic condition is wiped out, the fat inside the body is never again required, and dissolves away.

How To Lose Weight With Alkaline Food?

The body's the inside condition is somewhat alkaline,

which is the reason it requests a diet that is likewise marginally alkaline. The body's whole metabolic procedure relies upon a chemical situation. Our inner framework lives and bites the dust at the cell level, every one of the billions of cells that make up the human body is somewhat alkaline, and must keep up alkalinity to work and stay healthy and alive.

Alkaline Food will cause nourishment desires to die down usually because the acidity inside the inner condition is killed through the alkaline framing components. When the internal landscape is alkalized with alkaline water and essential nourishment as indicated by an alkaline diet (=weight loss diet), the body is allowed to discharge the acid waste and copies of fat. Along these lines, your pH level will likewise be adjusted, and each organ capacities better, supporting healthy digestion and making weight control a lot simpler.

Some Good Alkaline Foods

Crisp vegetables, greens, and grasses are the phenomenal enemy of yeast and against contagious nourishments, and green pastures, for example, grain or wheatgrass, are the absolute least calorie, most minimal sugar and most supplement rich food sources on earth (and contain high measures of fiber).

Alkaline nourishments are, for the most part, vegetables, particularly rough ones. Most alkalizing are wheat and horse feed grasses, new cucumber, and some sort of sprouts. Moreover, limes, tomatoes, and avocado additionally have an alkalizing impact on our body, the same as a general sort of seeds, tofu, new soybeans, almonds, or olive oil.

What Are The Results Of The Alkaline Diet?

When an alkaline diet is begun, the vast majority find that their pH usually turns out to be increasingly caustic. One gets the opportunity to perceive how particular kinds of dinners make an exceptionally acidic condition and figure out how to change their dietary patterns to more readily bolster weight control. At the point when pH balance is accomplished through essential nourishment and basic nutritional habits, the body drops typically to its healthy weight, nourishment longings will decrease, glucose levels are adjusted, and energy levels will increment monstrously.

So anyone prepared to seek after the way of better health, weight loss, and more energy ought to consider the upsides of the alkaline diet for accomplishing an ideal pH balance in the body. It is perfect for anybody anxious to fabricate an establishment for good health - presently and for the years to come. Equalization pH-Diet.com illuminates individuals about the over-acidification regarding the body because of quick-paced and unhealthy ways of life, which is the purpose behind numerous diseases and weight gain.

Alkaline Diet Can Save Your Life

The theory behind the alkaline diet is that because the pH of our body is somewhat salty, with an ordinary scope of 7.36 to 7.44, our food ought to mirror this and be marginally soluble. An unequal diet high in acidic nourishments like creature protein, caffeine, sugar, and handled nourishments will, in general, upset this equalization. It can drain the collection of alkaline minerals, for example, sodium, potassium, magnesium, and calcium, making individuals helpless against interminable and degenerative diseases.

Our inner concoction balance is fundamentally constrained by our lungs, kidneys, digestive organs, and skin. For fundamental capacities to happen, our body must keep up an appropriate pH. The proportion of the acidity or alkalinity of a substance is called pH. Sufficient alkaline stores are required for the ideal alteration of pH. The body needs oxygen, water, and acid-buffering minerals to achieve the pH-buffering while rapidly evacuating waste items.

The over-acidification of the body is the fundamental reason for all diseases. Soft drink is presumably the most acidic nourishment individuals expend at a pH of 2.5. Soft drink is multiple times more acidic than nonpartisan water and takes 32 glasses of impartial water to adjust a glass of pop. Alkaline nourishment and water ought to be devoured, to give supplements the body needs to kill acids and poisons from the blood, lymph, and tissues, and simultaneously, reinforces the safe and organ frameworks.

Most vegetables and organic products contain a higher measure of essential shaping components than different nourishments. The more noteworthy the ratio of green nourishments devoured in the diet, the more prominent the health benefits accomplished. These plant nourishments are purifying and alkalizing to the body, while the refined and handled nourishments can increment unhealthy degrees of acidity and poisons. Be that as it may, know that an excess of alkaline can likewise hurt you. You should have the best possible information on adjusting alkaline and acidic nourishments in your diet. After ingestion, alkaline nourishment and water are very quickly killed by hydrochloric acid present in the stomach. The harmony among alkaline and acidic nourishments must be kept up all together for your organs to perform well.

A healthy and adjusted diet is more alkaline than acid. Given your blood classification, the menu ought to be comprised of 60 to 80% alkaline nourishments and 20 to 40% acidic food sources. Typically, the A and AB blood classifications require the most alkaline diet, while the O and B blood classifications require creature items increasingly in their diet. In any case, remember, in case you're in torment, you're acidic. Progressing to an alkaline diet requires a move in one's mentality about nourishment. It is useful to investigate new tastes and surfaces while rolling out little improvements and improving old propensities.

How Alkaline Diet Recipes Whip Up Better Health

As a rule, this diet includes ingesting certain new citrus leafy foods that are low in sugar. It elevates to maintain a strategic distance from nourishment, which is high in acid, for example, grains, dairy, meat, sugar, liquor, caffeine, and parasites. It removes the day by day admission of acidic nourishments to the furthest reaches of 30% and lifts your alkaline access to 70%. The objective is to restrict or even dispense with the ingestion of nourishments, which are adverse to health and supplant it with delicious healthy alkaline diet recipes.

What are the models and impacts of acidic nourishment?

The present culture promotes moment and quick nourishments, and they are selling quickly, particularly for individuals who are consistently in a hurry. They will, in general, buy these greasy and high in sodium nourishment to augment their work time. Indeed, the promotions are phenomenal secrets to bait your hunger. One thing is, without a doubt, these prepared, bundled, and microwavable nourishments are directly harming our health upon ingestion the alkalinity of the blood focuses on the body controllers of acid-base homeostasis. Subsequently, drawn-out admission may result in losing the body's capacity to work well and even passing in some urgent cases.

Alkaline diet as a rule

The theory clarifies that after eating alkaline-rich nourishment, it leaves a chemical buildup or debris. Presently this debris is viewed as a mineral containing the chief components like calcium, iron, magnesium, copper, and zinc. These components add to keeping up the homeostasis of the body. Acidifying nourishments makes these essential minerals drop in levels inclining our body to different ailments connecting with too alkaline diet shields the body and keeps that from occurring. Fundamentally, our collection ought to keep up a pH of 7.3, which means to state, our body should be alkaline, and it ought to likewise reflect in our nourishment consumption. Alkaline diet doesn't merely shed the additional pounds off; however, well beyond that, it recaptures loss health and advances a long and without disease life.

Luring, perfect and delightful recipes to keep up an alkaline diet

Alkaline diet recipes incorporate a more elevated level of vegetable admission, a press of lemon into water drinks, millet or quinoa ought to supplant wheat and olive oil over vegetable oil, soups like miso best pursues the diet. Preparing a delicious lunch with a cucumber serving of mixed greens - the fixings are crisp tomatoes and cucumbers, balsamic vinegar, red wine, ocean salt, minced garlic, new basil and oregano, and additional virgin olive oil. For supper, you can make vegetable pasta with tomato-pepper sauce all you need is a vegetable or spelled pasta, sun-dried and new tomatoes, red ringer pepper, zucchini, onion and garlic, stew, fresh basil, cold-squeezed olive oil, and salt and pepper to taste (the vegetables are pan-seared and use it as a garnish to the pasta).

Presently, a supper would not be finished without a sweet, here are a portion of the irreproachable pastries that can fulfill your yearnings like crusty fruit-filled treat - you will require ground crude pecans, pitted dates absorbed alkaline water for 15 minutes, coarse sunflower seeds, destroyed apples, cinnamon, new squeezed apple, damaged coconut for decorating, and raisins or prunes. All the dry fixings, even the ones splashed and drained, ought to be blended in a nourishment processor and will fill in as the hull. For a snappier sweet, you can layer strawberries, blueberries, raspberries, blackberries, plain yogurt, and wheat germ and almonds for decorating a "berry" brilliant treat to be sure!

The Perks of the Alkaline Diet Program

Society today is assaulted by such a significant number of various diet programs that it very well may be overpowering. A few diets place limitations on what nourishments can be eaten due to what's in them, while others are progressively indulgent with nourishment determination, however stringent on when you can eat. The reason for diets differ too, and some are intended to get more fit and others are for improving health. The alkaline diet can be grouped into the last mentioned, as it comprises of expending healthy nourishments yet can at the previous outcome in weight loss too.

The pH level of the human body should be around 7.35, which is somewhat alkaline and implies that alkaline is required by the body. Trackers and gatherers, a long time prior, experienced no difficulty addressing this need as the vast majority of the nourishments they are were wealthy in alkaline, for example, vegetables, nuts, and seeds.

These days notwithstanding, the cutting edge diet isn't exceptionally alkaline, comprising mainly of handled nourishments and creature protein. At the point when these nourishments and different things, for example, espresso, beans, and fish, are expended, they discharge acids that happen to debilitate our bones.

The alkaline diet is engaging because it advances quality during the bones and joints. Acid debilitates the bones, so expending a diet high in alkaline will balance the impacts that acids have on our bodies. That is the reason this diet contains nourishments, for example, natural products, seeds, nuts, green tea, tomatoes, etc. because they have low degrees of acid. However, more grounded joints and bones aren't the main advantages of the alkaline diet.

Extra advantages of the alkaline diet incorporate expanded energy levels and hindering an abundance of mucous generation. It can likewise enable the individuals to experience the ill effects of this season's flu virus, colds, and nasal clog as often as possible. Also, the individuals who have different indications, for example, polycystic ovaries, ovarian pimples, and kindhearted bosom growths, can improve by changing to an alkaline-based diet. At last, it can decrease sentiments of crabbiness, uneasiness, and tension.

Alkaline Diet Chart

The alkaline acid is another diet that is increasing increasingly more prevalence. The menu depends on regular or all-encompassing mending methods and has been around for a long while. Recently, however, it has been picking up notoriety and not merely among health nuts. I chose to assemble an alkaline diet graph to show what nourishment is viewed as alkaline and healthful and which ones are viewed as acidic and ought to be kept away from!

Alkaline Diet Chart:

Profoundly Alkaline Foods According to the Alkaline Diet Chart

- Tangerine, Pineapple, Lotus Root, ocean salt,

lentils, Seaweed, watermelon, tangerine, preparing pop, onion, kelp, mineral water, sweet potato, lime, nectarine, persimmon, raspberry, pumpkin seeds, ocean vegetables

Decently Alkaline Foods as per the Alkaline Diet Chart

- kombucha, broccoli, grapefruit, melon, citrus, olive, loganberry, parsnip, unsulfured molasses, soy sauce, cashews, grapefruit, melon, honeydew, garlic, kale, parsley, endive, kohlrabi, chestnuts, pepper, mustard green, ginger, dewberry, arugula, olive

Low Alkaline Forming Foods According to the Alkaline Diet Chart

- Sesame seed, cherry, rutabaga, cauliflower, mu tea, rice syrup, almonds, blackberry, peach, ginseng, collard greens, rice syrup, papaya, cabbage, sharp apples, apple juice, mushrooms, avocado, chime pepper, potato, eggplant, grows, purpose, primrose, ringer pepper, apple juice vinegar

Exceptionally Low Alkaline Forming Foods According to the Alkaline Diet Chart

- celery, blueberry, raisin, wild rice, ghee, avocado oil, chive, most seeds, cilantro, currant, umeboshi vinegar, coconut oil, olive oil, duck eggs, cucumber, turnip greens, strawberry, flax oil, ghee, flax oil, beet, lettuces, banana, japonica rice, orange, Brussel grows, oats, grain espresso

Exceptionally Low Acid Forming Foods According to the Alkaline Diet Chart

- Alcohol, chard, plum, farina, elk, sheep, game mear, wheat, oil, lima beans, Teff, Kamut, flour, semolina, white rice, bovine milk, balsamic vinegar, milk, seitan, pinto beans, tofu, shellfish, lamb, dark tea, white rice, vanilla, naval force beans, pig, white beans, mollusks, buckwheat, almond oil, safflower, aduki beans, soy cheddar, shellfish, matured cheddar, tomatoes, red berries, sesame oil, aduki beans, almond oil

Respectably Acid Forming Foods According to the Alkaline Diet Chart

- Coffee, cranberry, walnuts, squid, maize, portion oil, corn, casein, milk protein, grease, oat grain, chicken, green peas, peanuts, pomegranate, soy milk, grain groats, cranberry, nutmeg, pistachios, chestnut oil, garbanzo beans, pork, mussels, rye, vegetables, veal

Profoundly Acid Forming nourishments to stay away from no matter what!!!

- pudding, seared nourishments, pecans, jam, sugars, brew, cola, pecans, hazelnuts, table salt, frozen yogurt, soybean, hamburger, bounces, malt, sodas, vinegar, prepared cheddar, lobster, sugar, grain, cottonseed oil, fowl.

Alkalizing Foods For The Alkaline Diet

The Alkaline diet is a diet that is intended to assist

you with accomplishing ideal health. The theory behind it is that the human body was designed to run Alkaline. Much the same as a vehicle is intended to run on gas. The body can run on acid; however, to do so, it will have invested time and a great deal of energy killing or adjusting that acid. The body does this by utilizing sodium bicarbonate or Baking Soda. The body takes sodium bicarbonate from your bones and different spots where it is expected to kill the acid and accomplish balance.

There are many alkalizing nourishments suggested for the alkaline diet. You are taking a gander at some of these to get a thought of what you ought to get a higher amount of in your alkaline diet. Alkalizing nourishments are nourishments that help to keep up alkalinity inside the blood.

Greens

Anything green will be beneficial for you. The darker the green, the higher the amount of alkalizing nourishment it is. Greens like spinach, kale, chard, collard, and dandelion will be the absolute most alkalizing nourishments. The more you eat, the better you will look and feel on the alkaline diet. I like to begin my day with a green smoothie. I take a lot of spinach, kale, and chard at that point mix everything up with some foods grown from the ground seeds and appreciate!

Grasses

Wheatgrass juice is by a wide margin one of the most alkalizing nourishments for the alkaline diet. This stuff is genuinely jam pressed with supplements. On an atomic level, wheatgrass is practically identical to the human blood. That just knocks my socks off. Wheatgrass contains each of the eight essential amino acids. It includes 13 other amino acids also. It is jam stuffed with nutrients, minerals, chlorophyll, and phytonutrients. If you are searching for alkalizing nourishments for the alkaline diet, look no further. Different grasses have comparable advantages of grain.

Sprouts

At the point when I initially began the alkaline diet, I was on a strict spending plan and couldn't bear the cost of a ton of nourishment. One thing that I began doing that I would suggest is developing my sprouts. Sprouts are another essential alkalizing nourishment for the alkaline diet. They are viewed as biogenic, which implies that the energy and quality of the plant developing from seed to grow are moved to the human body when you devour them. Sprouts can be expertly designed and added to your plates of mixed greens for the alkaline diet. Utilizing growing containers, you can without much of a stretch increase a considerable amount of sprouts in as meager as 5-7 days. My undisputed top choice sprouts are broccoli sprouts, and horse feed grows. I am likewise inclined toward mung bean grows.

Water

Water, water, water, and afterward, more water. Drinking heaps of water is incredibly bravo and can likewise help in alkalizing the body. I did a test as of late. I went to a characteristic stream close to my home at a high rise. I topped off a water bottle. I returned home and tried the PH of the water. It was incredibly alkaline water. I, at that point, continued to test the PH of the water I regularly drink, which is switch assimilation water from a neighborhood water organization. This water was acidic.

CHAPTER FOUR
DETOXING THE LIVER

The liver is a significant organ that ought to be given appropriate consideration. Its job is to get out poisons from the body. Looking at the situation objectively, it is overpowering what number of toxins get into our bodies every day. Each time an individual eats something unhealthy drinks, an excessive amount of liquor consumes medications or smokes, toxins are ingested. Every one of these poisons is handled by the liver that, at that point, puts forth a valiant effort to get these poisons out of the body through an individual's pee, fecal matter, or sweat.

In any case, the liver has its points of confinement. Now and again, the liver gets over-burden and can't process the poisons out of an individual's framework. This can have grievous ramifications for an individual's health. It is significant for an individual to do all that is in their capacity to keep the liver working great. Going on a liver detox diet now and then can assist the liver with clearing out overabundance poisons and remain in high working request.

Various liver diets are drifting around. One can discover a diet of this nature online effectively. A few foods just last a couple of days while others last as long as three weeks. Most liver detox diets comprise of eating generally uncooked products of the soil alongside entire grain nourishments. Water additionally assumes a significant job in any liver detox diet. An individual that is going on such a diet should drink in any event eight cups of water every day for it to be mighty. Low-quality nourishments handled nourishments, liquor, espresso, and drugs must be surrendered while going on a liver detox diet.

The Seven Day Liver Detox Diet Plan:

Day 1-Day 3: This period of this diet includes drinking just fluids. An individual that sets out on this specific diet should confine oneself to just drinking new lime squeeze and loads of water. This stage is one of the most troublesome, as an individual is fundamentally fasting and will feel feeble and tired. One can, on the off chance that the person wants, do some light exercise while on this period of the liver detox diet. Be that as it may, it is essential to enable a lot of time to rest and not exaggerate.

Day 4 - Day 6: This period of the liver detox diet is a lot simpler to deal with. An individual can eat every homemade food grown from the ground. Entire grain nourishments and bubbled vegetables are additionally permitted. Nonetheless, while an individual can eat certain nourishments at this phase of the detox diet, the person in question will likewise need to keep on drinking a lot of fluids. Fluids that are allowed at this phase of the menu are juices, homegrown teas, and handcrafted products of the soil juice.

Day 7: One can eat similar nourishments that are taken into account days 4 - 6. One can likewise steam their vegetables as opposed to eating them either crude or bubbled. Herbs that are prescribed for this phase of the diet are Rosemary and Dandelion.

While going on a liver detox diet is an extraordinary method to enable the liver to wipe out poisons from the framework, it can likewise have negative symptoms. An individual ought to counsel their PCP before setting out on this kind of purging. A person that was encountering indications, for example, retching and agony, should stop the diet promptly and look for medicinal assistance.

The most effective method to Cleanse Your Liver

One of the significant organs of the body is the liver. For individuals who keep up a functioning way of life that incorporates liquor and utilization of specific nourishments, these individuals may need to do some liver detox. One may ask, what is liver detox? The appropriate response is straightforward. It is the straightforward procedure of eating nourishment that is useful for the liver and drinking water for in any event seven days. This will begin the liver detox procedure of the liver and would empower it to carry out its responsibility well once more. Like different things, the liver, alongside different organs in the body, must not be mishandled. It is regular information that everything in overabundance is risky and abusing the liver, the body, and considerably different organs for quite a while will clearly introduce some health issues en route. Another extraordinary expansion to the recipe for organization and liver purging is natural dandelion cases. These are accessible on health stores, staple goods, and drug stores. The homegrown dandelion cases flush the poisons of the body and enable the liver to recoup quicker.

Inside the liver is the bile; this is the piece of the liver that isolates the fats and cholesterol from the nourishment individuals eat. The bile is essential to keep the digestive tract healthy and to dodge the stoppage. During the time spent liver detox, one of the most supportive fixings is the milk thorn seed extricate. Other nourishment that is vital in the liver detox diet is garlic, green vegetables, olive oil, grapefruit, cabbage, beets and carrots, avocados, lemons and limes, entire grains, and cruciferous vegetables including broccoli, kale, and cauliflower. Extra nourishment that is extraordinary for the detox diet is apples, whole grains, complete nuts, asparagus, and so on.

For individuals who need to realize how to cleanse your liver, here is a straightforward rule.

- Before: Avoid nourishment and drinks with destructive poisons, for example, caffeine, sugar, unpure water, liquor, and artificial sugars.

- During: Liquid diet on the initial two days; natural products, steamed vegetables, and steamed rice on the following four days; and expansion of other liver-accommodating nourishment on a diet.

- After: Return to ordinary diet, however, cut out on unhealthy nourishment and refreshments like bundled food sources, refined nourishments, low-quality nourishments, wheat, eggs, sugar, and other handled food sources. Likewise, it is significant in liver detox to diminish the utilization of caffeine, liquor, tobacco, and road drugs.

There are numerous ways on the most proficient method to detox your body, and in spite of the fact that it very well may be exceptionally testing, it isn't really inconceivable. Vital nourishment for the liver detox is as of now referenced previously. Make sure to remember that nourishment for the day by day diet and drink loads of water each day. Liver detox is an incredible method to filter the liver from every one of the poisons present in the body. If the liver gets exhausted and an individual neglects to detox his/her liver, the liver may all of a sudden separate and discharge a pool of smelling salts into the blood. This is hazardous and can prompt the severe harm of the sensory system, liver, mind, and kidneys. The body may likewise discharge lactic acid, which can cause constant weariness, hurting muscles, cerebral pain, tension, alarm assaults, and hypertension.

Step by step instructions to Start a Liver Detox Diet

A healthy liver can be acquired with the best possible measure of the correct sort of diet. The liver purging diet is presently a need in the general public because most nourishment that individuals eat nowadays contains additives and fake added substances that are significant for long stockpiling period yet destructive for our liver. To have a productive and successful liver purging diet, you should begin the correct way. So how are we going to start our liver purging food?

Before beginning a liver detoxification diet, make an agenda on the side effects (hypersensitivities, stench, nervousness, asthma, swelling, hypertension, low blood method, cold feet and hands, desires, stoppage, misery, looseness of the bowels, dry hair, dry skin, low energy, unpredictable glucose, weight addition, peevishness, and others) that you are presently encountering. Screen your body once per month to note if your body has come back to its best condition. It is additionally useful to make a rundown of nourishment that you expend to figure out what food should be dispensed with and what is to be kept up.

Seven days before the beginning of executing your

liver purifying diet, you should quit smoking and drinking mixed drinks to avert over-burdening the liver that may cause trouble in wiping out harmful squanders that have gathered our body. Additionally, have a healthy diet by taking up crisp products of the soil and lessen the utilization of nourishments with a high measure of additives and other prepared food sources. Recollect that enormous numbers of the nourishments we expend every day contain unnatural poisons, for example, cancer-causing agents, anti-infection agents, pesticides, hormone medications, and fake sugars that may harm our liver.

Body condition is fundamental before a liver purging detox. Significantly, your body is decidedly ready to take a detox since you won't be permitted to devour healthy nourishments during a detox diet. It is additionally prudent to examine with your doctor the liver detox plan that you are going to take to evade different inconveniences to happen. Legitimate exercise will likewise have a molded body when a detox diet.

Light fasting seven days before your purging diet can be beneficial. The light diet contains heaps of water, crisp organic product juices, raw vegetables, and new natural products. New nourishments include more compounds that are fundamental in your liver purging diet. It additionally makes sure to eat at the correct time to abstain from overemphasizing your liver during the body molding. When your body is adapted, the danger of encountering undesirable reactions will be diminished.

Body detoxification can be begun with lessening your utilization of nourishments that has a high amount of poisons, for example, prepared food sources, liquor, artificial sugar, and espresso and increment your measure of admission of new leafy foods.

How Important is Your Liver's Health in Weight Management?

How significant is it to have a healthy liver when following a weight loss program?

• Nonalcoholic fatty liver disease is, at present, the most widely recognized liver disease around the world.

• All phases of nonalcoholic greasy liver disease are presently accepted to be because of insulin obstruction, a condition intently connected with heftiness.

• Tests show that in individuals with liver issues, the higher an individual's BMI (Body Mass Index), the more prominent the liver harm.

Perhaps the best worry in this nation is obesity in children. Furthermore, wouldn't you know it, so is youth NAFLD (Nonalcoholic Fatty Liver Disease).

Losing abundance weight is the foundation of the treatment of nonalcoholic greasy liver disease. There are meds that specialists can use to treat NAFLD; however, shedding pounds through diet and exercise is as yet the absolute best treatment. Nonetheless, this might be quite difficult. We live in a general public where high-fat, high carbohydrate, unhealthy nourishments are the standard, and exercise is an exertion. Diabetes is a scourge, and it is evaluated that 90% of individuals with Type 2 diabetes have greasy liver disease.

Insulin Resistance is the most significant contributing component of stoutness. Stomach fat is the snitch story indication of Insulin Resistance. How would you look? You may require some assistance, yet diabetes and weight increase can be overseen. At last, advancing healthy dietary patterns and a functioning way of life, particularly in children, will most completely counteract NAFLD (greasy liver disease) and Type 2 diabetes.

Greasy liver in itself is nothing to stress over and will vanish with loss of weight. The ideal approach to test is through a straightforward blood test to check whether liver chemicals come back to ordinary after weight loss. If they do, you can be quite well sure NAFLD (nonalcoholic greasy liver disease) was the issue. In any case, to be satisfied, solitary a liver biopsy can tell, which is costly and nosy, and for the most part, not worth the dangers.

At the point when Fatty Liver is left untreated, it forms into steatohepatitis, a condition where fat is amassed in the liver; however, there is irritation (hepatitis). Liver cell passes on (putrefaction) and scarring (fibrosis) happen. Fibrosis of the liver would then be able to advance to cirrhosis of the liver, which is the last phase of nonalcoholic greasy liver disease.

Perhaps the ideal approach to secure against insulin opposition is to keep up a healthy liver in any case. Bile that is created in the liver is the thing that uses fat cells. On the off chance that the liver is working appropriately and isn't poisonous and exhausted, it will play out its weight the executives work effectively, and you won't need to endeavor to keep the lbs off.

Artichoke and Sarsaparilla are an incredible mix of liver health.

Artichoke improves liver capacity, including bile generation for fat digestion; Increases the excellent HDL cholesterol; Lowers raised blood lipids, cholesterol and triglycerides; and Detoxes the liver and different organs of the body.

Sarsaparilla cleanses the blood, helps in bladder health and hormone balance in the two people.

Look at it. It is anything but a regular thing. On more than one occasion per year should keep most everyone's liver running right. Particularly on the off chance that they are eating right and practicing and not manhandling their liver with broad liquor utilization.

Control your weight and secure your liver

simultaneously. Your health may rely upon it.

If you or somebody you realize has over the top tummy fat, truly consider NAFLD. This impacts children just as grown-ups and may require prompt consideration. It is anything but difficult to turn around when gotten early.

Outside Toxins and the Effect They Have on the Liver

We have seen the need to eat nourishments that will help detox the liver, and how infrequent liver detoxification to flush poisons out of the framework is useful. In any case, how would we maintain a strategic distance from these poisons in any case? You may be acquainted with a panic that has turned into a web sensation over the harmful impact of a vehicle's cooling framework; there is a considerable amount of disinformation out there also. I won't go into it here, yet teaching yourself on every one of these issues will assist you with expelling these bits of gossip.

In any case, it is evident that we all, and particularly those with persistent liver disease, ought to be wary against significant levels of natural poisons. A portion of the manners in which we can have more noteworthy genuine feelings of serenity to lessen our introduction to toxins are:

1. Maintain a strategic distance from all tobacco

smoke. By not smoking, yet evade all recycled smoke too. The vast majority comprehend the harm tobacco smoke can do to the heart and lungs. However, it likewise negatively affects the liver. The poisons in smoke lead to constant aggravation and scarring in the liver cells, which can prompt cancer and liver fibrosis.

Another intriguing reality about how tobacco smoke influences the liver is how it manages nicotine, the most addictive fixing in cigarettes. At the point when you breathe in this nicotine, the liver produces compounds to sift these poisons through as more nicotine comes into the body, the more catalysts that will be created by the liver to free yourself of the destructive poisons. This may appear to be something worth being thankful for. However, it just adds to the dependence, as the body wants more nicotine to stay aware of what it loses because of the expanded compound generation. That is the reason what used to fulfill a smoker's longings never again works, and a pack a day transforms into a few.

2. Farthest point gas smolder presentation. Those vapor indeed are terrible for you. The liver will evacuate these poisons, yet on the off chance that severely strained, the liver may become overpowering. Much will rely upon the length and power of the presentation, yet the more that can be stayed away from, the better. There are filling stations now that have fume recuperation frameworks to catch the exhaust. This incorporates maintaining a strategic distance from gas contacting

your skin.

3. Comprehend that benzene-containing synthetic compounds are unsafe. You can smell them with solvents, artistry supplies, and paints. This is frequently because of benzene, which is a lethal synthetic that can add to an over-burden of liver danger. It used to be utilized as an added substance to gas, yet has been diminished in ongoing decades. On the off chance that you must associate with items that contain benzene, be sure the region is all around ventilated.

4. Breathing in exhaust vapor can be dangerous. On the off chance that you are sitting in rush hour gridlock, there might be little you can do to abstain from breathing these exhaust. One choice is to hold the windows down and change your vehicle's ventilation framework to re-course. There will, at present, be some poisonous vapor in this air, yet positively not almost to the degree the outside fumes exhaust from sitting vehicles.

Restoring Fibroids Naturally - The Role Played by Detoxing the Liver

There are different components contained inside a fruitful arrangement for relieving fibroids usually, and powerful liver detox is a fundamental piece of any great framework. Keeping up a healthy liver is significant for good, generally speaking, health, yet on the off chance that you are inclined to fibroids, at that point, it is totally essential that your liver is in the best of health.

The liver is liable for creating different substances, which are essential for the health of the resistant framework, keeping up hormonal parity and glucose levels, and adding to our fruitfulness. It additionally assumes a vital job in helping expel infections, yeasts, and flotsam and jetsam from the body. On the off chance that your liver isn't working appropriately, this can prompt hormonal unevenness, the poor working of the safe framework, and insulin obstruction, all of which add to the development of fibroids.

There are five components to consider for an effective liver detox which will help in relieving fibroids usually:-

1. Eat a low-fat diet wealthy in nuts, beans, seeds, and non-bland vegetables. Incorporate garlic and onions, however, maintain a strategic distance from refined carbohydrates, hydrogenated oils, liquor, and soaked fats

2. Take a decent, all-around multivitamin and mineral enhancement

3. A juice quick will help with liver detoxification and help to flush out lethal mixes

4. Take the enhancements, Milk Thistle, Chlorine, and Betaine-all of which help to help the liver

5. Direct a Liver Flush

Albeit a liver detox is just a single piece of a general arrangement for restoring fibroids; usually, it is an essential part and ought not to be disregarded. Different components incorporate finding a way to change your diet and exercise levels and stress the executives.

Does Lemon Juice Detox the Liver?

The liver is a crucial organ that can't be supplanted by any type of mechanical gear. The numerous jobs that our liver plays in our body incorporate hormone generation, glycogen stockpiling, digestion, and above all, detoxification. Numerous individuals, who endeavor detoxification frequently wonder, does lemon juice detox the liver? The lemon detox diet plan is a notable arrangement that is intended to cleanse your liver. Aside from health aficionados, numerous ladies take up the lemon detox diet aim to help them with getting in shape.

A lemon detox diet plan is necessary and helpful. The drink comprises madalbal tree syrup, water, ocean salt, cayenne pepper, and in conclusion, lemons. The madalbal tree syrup is a syrup that contains five diverse tree saps. This syrup is concoction and additive-free.

Does lemon juice detox the liver?

Lemon's new squeeze is equipped for helping our stomach digest the supplements that our body gets for the day. Additionally, crisp lemon juice goes about as a cell reinforcement. As a significant aspect of the citrus family, lemon juice contains high measures of nutrient C. Things being what they are, how can it help with detoxification of the liver?

Lemon juice goes about as a filtration framework in your body. Lemon juice keeps unpalatable supplements from entering your bloodstream. This enables your liver to take a break from its filtration work — high measures of nutrient C, which is a cancer prevention agent.

Lemons contain high measures of nutrient C, which functions as a cancer prevention agent. The nutrients C present in fruits is equipped for evacuating free radicals that are created by your liver when it channels your circulatory system. Cell reinforcements are provided for killing free radicals.

Increment Of Bile stream

The point of a liver detox is to expel poisons from your liver. This should be possible by expanding the bile stream. Bile is a liquid that is delivered by your liver. The capacity of bile is to provide related stomach juice and to wipe out specific substances from your body via completing them of your body as excretion. Lemon juice builds the generation of bile by your liver. In the wake of perusing the accompanying advantages that lemon juice can accomplish for your liver, you should know whether lemon juice detoxes the liver. Try not to depend exclusively on this refreshment for liver detox.

Increment your utilization of new foods grown from the ground to keep your liver healthy!

Nourishments That Detox The Liver And Remove Cellulite

Cellulite is the orange strip-like appearance of fat on the skin, generally starting on the thighs, at that point progressing to different pieces of the body. Practically 85% of ladies have cellulite; in any case, whether they are fat or thin, youthful or old. Luckily, there are nourishments that detox the liver and help lessen the presence of the horrible appearance of the skin.

How Does Liver Detoxification Help?

At the point when the liver is exhausted or unhealthy, it can't viably manage the female estrogen that is thought to contribute to the advancement of cellulite. Anything that ruins legitimate dissemination of lymphatic liquid or blood can cause skin issues. Different components that likewise add to this are the absence of activity, lacking water consumption, extreme pressure, unhealthy eating, obstruction, hormonal cycles, weak breathing, and air contamination. The liver needs to work always in managing poisons noticeable all around, on what you apply on your skin, and so on. If it can't deal with every one of those things, cellulite will show up. In this way, purifying the liver will significantly help in facilitating the poisons that have aggregated during its sifting capacities in the body.

Apples

They are wealthy in gelatin, an intricate type of carbohydrate that is required by the body in purging and taking out poisons from your stomach related tract. Eating an apple daily will give your liver a simpler time in taking care of the grievous burden it needs to channel.

Avocado

This is another super nourishment that is thick in supplements that advance the body in creating glutathione compounds required by the liver to sift through poisons from the lymphatic liquids and blood successfully.

Beets, Carrots

The two vegetables are wealthy in beta-carotene and plant flavonoids that will animate, just as improve elements of the liver.

Garlic

This herb can make dinners delicious; however, that isn't the chief marvel it can do. Garlic offers a lot of health benefits, and among them is that it can actuate liver proteins to flush out poisons from the body. It additionally contains selenium and allicin, exacerbates that likewise help cleanse the organ.

Grapefruit

This organic product contains high measures of cancer prevention agents and nutrient C, which both assistance improve the standard liver purifying capacities. Press your cut grapefruit to fill a little glass with a new squeeze. Drink it up to lift liver protein creation. With this, poisons and cancer-causing agents can be effectively flushed out.

Green Tea

It contains catechins, plant cancer prevention agents, or aggravate that guides liver generation. This reviving tea can likewise improve your general health and aid your weight loss objectives.

Green Leafy Vegetables

These vegetables can be eaten cooked, crude, or squeezed. They can supply you with loads of plant chlorophyll that can sufficiently siphon poisons in your circulation system. These supplements rich vegetables can kill synthetic concoctions, substantial metals, and pesticides; therefore, offering incredible assurance for the organ. Join green and verdant vegetables in your diet, for example, spinach, mustard, and severe gourd in your dinners. This will build bile creation, and stream so squanders can be successfully expelled from the blood and the organs.

Lemons, Limes

Fresh lemon juice can offer a lot of health benefits, mostly blood filtering and weight loss.

Detox Your Liver in 7 Days With A Liver Detox Diet

Among the diverse body parts, the liver is among one of the significant organs, for it has considerable capacity in body detoxification. Through this body detoxification, synthetics and other outside substances like poisons and even defecation, pee, and sweat are expelled from the body. These substances originate from the unsafe nourishments that we eat like handled and non-regular rich nourishments, liquor drinks that we devour, cigarettes that we smoke, and even drugs that we expend for anti-infection treatment and hormone elective drugs. These substances are the ones that our bodies attempt to take out every day.

When there are many harming materials inside the body, the liver needs to keep keeping up until its ability runs out. When this is dismissed, vast amounts of poisons can be gathered in the body and will cause many body issues and diseases. To anticipate this and keep up excellent health, we should experience a detoxification diet and take significant consideration of our liver.

A liver detoxification plan can be completed either on a three-day, seven-day, or twenty-one-day program. This depends on a firm focus on a diet with unprocessed and natural foods grown from the ground, entire grains, and water cure with enough measure of water or liquid other option. Nourishments that are wealthy in fat or sugar, caffeine, liquor drinks, unnatural and human-made nourishment, drugs, and low-quality nourishments would all be able to must be put to a stop, at any rate, seven days before the diet plan.

The Seven Day Liver Detoxification Diet

One to Three Days: This is the period to start your fluid diet plan where you need to drink around ten to twelve glasses of water ordinarily alongside frequently crushed lime juice. Even though it can indeed be challenging to execute this diet because of the weariness and slightness, light exercise can be included as a request to affix the method of flushing the poisons out of the body. Additionally, you should shun taking in any sort of milk or dairy item.

Four to Six Days: Fresh organic products, vegetables, and entire grains can be expended like celery, apples, carrots, oranges, which would all be able to be blended into one juice. The juice can incorporate your selection of leafy foods. Even though healthy nourishments are devoured, there are as yet liquid choices, for example, natural teas for around a few cups every day. Concerning suppers, they can incorporate cut and bubbled vegetables like celery, carrots, broccoli, and spinach. Besides, you can likewise utilize soups that can be taken in at regular intervals.

Seven days: Along with the leafy foods, the liquids are expended together. They would all be able to be arranged by having them crude or steamed. Additionally, you can consume rosemary tea and dandelion options, which can be useful for this period.

You can generally change the sorts of foods grown from the ground that you will use as long as you oblige the strategy. When the seventh day is a doe, you can participate in the typical diet; finally, however, there is still a restriction on liquor consumption for around one entire week after the detoxification diet. You have to end the food once you feel torment, disorder, and squeamishness. Most likely, this detoxification diet can have an enormous impact on the advancement and support of a healthy lifestyle.

Instructions to Detox Your Body With Alternative Therapies

Conventional Chinese Medicine (TCM) is a fantastic asset when figuring out how to detox your body, and is mainly prescribed for treating stomach related issue, for example, bad-tempered inside syndrome; ceaseless skin conditions like dermatitis; weariness and despair; hormonal awkward nature, for example, PMS; endometriosis and poor sperm tally, and barrenness (both male and female). It can create results with interminable conditions that Western methods neglect to help. At the point when joined with a detox diet, it can make perceptible upgrades to a people's health and prosperity.

Self-finding and treatment of ailments are not suggested; however, at some TCM focuses, you can portray your side effects to the specialist behind the counter and get a suitable cure on the spot. TCM can be useful for treating individuals experiencing withdrawal from drug and liquor addictions. Liquor makes liver and nerve bladder uneven characters, which realizes a mix of unnecessary moistness and warmth.

Numerous drugs are prepared through the liver, making it warmed and blocked, so the liver's blood gets frail and insufficient. TCM equations center on clearing and supporting the liver and nerve bladder, while simultaneously treating the heart, to help quiet the brain and sensory system. Consolidating TCM with figuring out how to detox your body yourself is probably the best thing you can accomplish for your health.

Ayurvedic Body Detox Techniques

Ayurveda is an old Indian arrangement of health care, and, similar to Chinese prescription, it depends on balance inside the body. There are three essential doshas - Kapha, pitta, and Vata - of which we as a whole have various degrees in our bodies and characters, and treating side effects of un-health will include adjusting the doshas. A detox diet is simply part of this framework that you can pursue alone or as a significant aspect of a general body purifying methodology.

Ayurveda is a finished all-encompassing framework that should just be pursued under the supervision of a certified specialist. The fundamental method of detoxification, which is called Panchakarma, chips away at a few levels. To begin with, your diet is gotten out and purging nourishments. For example, Richard (produced using basmati rice, mung beans, and vegetables) are prescribed. Natural liver detox supplements are given to cleanse the inside and flush out poisons from the liver, blood, sweat organs, and skin. These will be explicitly structured by your dosha balance. You might be given a back rub with natural oils, heat treatment to open the circulatory channels, and bowel purges.

The most effective method to Detox Your Body WithNasya

It is also called nose purifying, and this is a piece of Ayurvedic body detox that numerous individuals have known about. It includes flushing a cured oil through the nose and sinuses, in one nostril and out the other, to cleanse poisons from the head and neck. Results can be set apart for the individuals who experience the ill effects of cerebral pains and headache, nasal hypersensitivities, sinusitis, poor memory or visual perception, and certain neurological conditions.

Advantages

Late trial of Ayurvedic body detox diet procedures at the University of Colorado found that the individuals who had experienced a few detoxes had lower levels of PCBs, DDT, and pesticide buildups than the benchmark group altogether.

It had all the earmarks of being especially powerful on fat-dissolvable poisons of the sort related to hormone interruption, concealment of the invulnerable framework, hypersensitivities, and diseases of the liver and skin. If there is a decent Ayurvedic facility close to you, it could merit doing an Ayurvedic body detox.

Some correlative scientific experts stock surely understood Ayurvedic cures that they could prescribe to treat singular manifestations. However, a total Panchakarma body detox must be done under expert supervision.

The most effective method to Detox Your Body Naturally

Figuring out how to detox your body [can have a significant effect on your health and prosperity. We are assaulted with poisons at consistently expanding rates from the air we inhale and the nourishment we eat. So following a healthy detox diet program at regular intervals is turning out to be progressively significant consistently. Begin today.

Herbs That Detox the Body - The Top 5 Herbs That Detox the Body Quickly

Everybody realizes that it is so critical to detox your body usually, supposing that you don't then poisons develop and this can have transient consequences for you, for example, tiredness, laziness, and absence of energy and even some long haul impacts, for example, expanded danger of specific disease.

There is a lot of costly detox medicines accessible. Yet, little to individuals realize that the absolute best detox specialists are exceptionally modest and can be found in your ordinary market or store. These herbs that detox the body are beneficial for your body and won't just assist it with detoxing; however will likewise give you better by and abundant health, expanded energy, and a more grounded safe framework.

All in all, what are the best herbs that detox the body?

I have gathered the accompanying rundown of top 5 herbs that will indeed fortify your body's detox motor and will assist you with detoxing substantially more rapidly on the off chance that you consolidate them into your diet:

1.) Burdock

This is incredible for detoxing; burdock attaches truly help to decrease the development of substantial metals in your framework, which won't just cleanse your arrangement of these undesirable poisons, yet will diminish the danger of safe framework issues later on.

2.) Nettles

Sounds frightful, I know, yet Nettles have some extremely extraordinary detox properties. One of the principle preferences of this herb is that it will cleanse your urinary framework and will counteract any future issues happening.

3.) Milk Thistle

Of the considerable number of herbs that detox the body, this one is most likely one of only a handful, not many that truly helps protein combination in your liver. It will fortify this procedure and make it work considerably more productively.

4.) Dandelion

Dandelion pulls are incredible cleansers for your nerve bladder and liver and will keep them healthy and clean.

5.) Psyllium Seeds

These seeds advance healthy solid discharges and guarantee that everything stays working effectively. This is one of only a handful of scarcely any herbs that detox the body that demonstrations like a kind of wipe and truly helps to wipe up undesirable poisons before being expelled from the body.

For what reason Do We Need To Detox The Body?

Detoxification is turning out to be increasingly more significant as time passes by, there are 300,000 new poisons/polluting influences compromising the body every year. That is 6,000 per week that are being added to the Chemical Society's Chemical Abstract. These poisons, some undeniable and some covered up, are making our bodies acidic. In an acidic domain, the disease develops and spreads, anything from the regular cold to cancer contingent upon how poisonous/acidic your body is.

These poisons are surrounding us, it is anything but an instance of escaping from them which would be virtually unimaginable except if you secured yourself a cleaned hatchery, yet monitoring them and decreasing the sum you open your body to these harming synthetic concoctions. Alright, so were all mindful of certain poisons, for example, liquor, smoking, drugs, carbon dioxide noticeable all around we breathe, and so forth. However, the dangerous ones are the ones we didn't even know we were expending, i.e.;

Medicine - solution, and non-physician endorsed drugs are risky, and inside the body become an exceptionally poisonous acid, making the body progressively acidic; the more acidic you are, the more defenseless against disease you become.

Water - The water we drink contains chlorine....but chlorine is utilized to kill living beings in our pools; last time I looked, we were a living being? Likewise, ongoing investigations propose to have discovered antidepressants and conception prevention drug in the water we drink.

Skin - Nobody likes to smell, however, in the antiperspirant and antiperspirants we use is a concoction called aluminum cholorohydrate, which is legitimately connected with bosom cancer, to such a degree, that numerous produces have prohibited this from being utilized and gone for the more "characteristic" way!

Diet items - One of the most significant misinterpretations is that "diet" items assist us with getting more fit when everything they do is make us fatter and progressively dangerous. In diet soft drinks, for instance, the ordinary sugar utilized in standard items has been taken out yet lamentably been supplanted with a compound turning out to be increasingly more well-known called Aspartame (there are more than 92 distinctive health indications related with aspartame) which is multiple times better than sugar. At 86 °f, aspartame is separated into another compound formaldehyde. The temperature of the body is 98.6 degrees Fahrenheit! Formaldehyde is utilized as a treating specialist who prevents the body from deteriorating; Formaldehyde can arrive in a glass holder alongside a significant red sign saying DANGER!!

Nourishment - The number of inhabitants on the planet is expanding a seemingly endless amount of time after a year, putting nourishment organizations/ranchers compelled to deliver more nourishment and speedier and with a more drawn out rack life......when was the last time you saw your milkman?? We use to get fresh milk delivered each morning; however, now the milk will last as long as seven days. Why? The additives put in our nourishment give it a more extended timeframe of realistic usability because there is such a significant amount of rivalry for our custom added substances are utilized to get you dependent on that specific brand, we as a whole know the motto for Pringles... "When you pop.. You can't stop" you will pop if you don't stop!! The nourishment we presently expend would one say one is of the most awkward things to our health; we can get an entire supper that can be kept for a year and afterward prepared in a short time?? How does that work, Nutritional value. Zero! We are eating extraordinary nourishment to what our folks ate and what their people ate. As the nature of food has disintegrated throughout the year's disease has been on the expansion.

Stress - When the body is focused on climate, physical, mental, or enthusiastic, it discharges a hormone called cortisol. Cortisol is a poison to the collection and builds fat stockpiling by expanding your hunger for high fat and high carbohydrate nourishments, and you become a thick putting away machine when focused. Cortisol debilitates your resistant framework by making your body progressively acidic and leaving you increasingly vulnerable to disease.

So to separate it, the more poisons you take in, the more acidic you become, and the more acidic you are, the almost certain you are to get cancer! Detox intends to dispose of poisons. The body detoxifies typically itself. Still, since of the measure of poisons, the body takes in the liver which is the primary detoxifying organ in the body battles to adapt and only like a shower when it's full, and the tap is as yet running the poisons flood into the body causing acidic/harmful situations. Our body's normal PH levels are 7.34, but since of the measure of poisons, we are presented to our bodies to move into an acidic state regularly. As you most likely are aware, now in an acidic domain, microscopic organisms and disease will develop.

The body's characteristic guard is to clutch any water that you take in to adjust the acid/alkaline levels, causing an additional couple of pounds of water maintenance. The measure of times I've heard individuals state, "On the off chance that I could simply lose two or three pounds," There most likely clutching 5lbs of water maintenance given the poisons they store in the body...

Recall the poisons we take in are an acid; because

were taking it in limited quantities, it doesn't mean it's not seriously affecting our health. Sadly when we have been determined to have something is the point at which we begin to respond to it. I generally state be PRO dynamic, not RE dynamic. So how would we do it, we need the most alkaline characteristic enhancements that are accessible to us;

Stage 1 in our healthy starter packs, we utilize natural herbs like psyllium structures, burdock, dark pecan, cascara, blackthorn, gentian and peony, and others to detox the body and dispose of all the danger that has developed inside you. This will detox your liver, kidneys, colon, and fat stores that store poisons. This will keep going for ten days; you will consider changes to be ahead of schedule as the third or fourth day.

Stage 2 to be done simultaneously and proceeded after the initial multi day's is to fuse fluid chlorophyll, chlorophyll advances the natural purifying elements of the body, reinforces cells, and freshens up the body, including the bowl.

Blend 1 teaspoon (5ml) liquid chlorophyll with water twice every day. Notwithstanding its extraordinary mending properties, chlorophyll is nontoxic and incredible for the entire family to utilize.

Stage 3, after the underlying ten days of taking acidity out, were going to return in great microorganisms to secure us, and this comes as acidophilus, which is usually found inside the intestinal tract, however, poisons and prescription wipe these out. Each case gives 3.5 billion advantageous microbes to the body. Two containers to be taken twice day by day.

This extremely viable detox can be made significantly progressively feasible whenever pursued by our natural detox diet.

Detoxing benefits;

- Increased energy
- Weight loss and increment indigestion
- Clearer skin and improved complexion
- Improved insusceptible framework
- Increased fixation
- Improved absorption
- Strengthens the body's battle against cancer cells and produces healthy cells
- Purify the blood
- Cellulite decrease

Different organs that get detoxed incorporate the kidneys, circulation system, colon, lymphatic framework, thrusts, and skin. Recall detoxing your bodies resembles taking your vehicle for assistance, and how frequently do you do that?

The Alkaline Diet and Acidosis

An alkaline diet is a diet-dependent on the ph scale. It originates from the Latin "pondus hydro genii." In English, this is genuinely Hydrogen Power or Hydrogen Potential. It is a proportion of the focus $H3O+$ of in arrangement science. The pace of cell metabolic movement influences and, simultaneously, is influenced by the pH of the body liquids. In warm-blooded creatures, the average pH of blood vessel blood lies somewhere in the range of 7.35 and 7.50 relying upon the species (for example, healthy human-blood vessel blood pH differs somewhere in the field of 7.35 and 7.45). Blood pH esteems perfect with life in well-evolved creatures are constrained to a pH go somewhere in the range of 6.8 and 7.8. Changes in the pH of blood vessel blood (and subsequently the extracellular liquid) outside this range bring about irreversible cell harm.

Well, the human body was worked to address ph issues. Throughout the years, our condition has developed increasingly lethal. Private enterprise has made nourishment makers do everything without exception in their influence to mass-produce food sources to get more cash-flow. This, as well as we have progressed in the course of the most recent 100 years from eating home developed or privately developed regular nourishment to eating god realizes what at taco chime and McDonald's. 90% of the populace doesn't have a clue what they are eating is unsafe. They expend prepared nourishment that has headed out miles and miles to get to the supermarket. Our bodies have reached so immersed with acids, that they can never again address the issue. So what occurs? Our bodies accomplish a detail of Acidosis.

What Is Acidosis?

Acidosis is by and large found in medication as a component of the pathology of a couple of various diseases, for example, debilitated liver capacity. It is experienced off and on again and even considered to by typical. Acidosis is unquestionably not typical. Some state that is the starter, if not the reason for persistent degenerative diseases. These incorporate cancer, diabetes, joint inflammation, and coronary illness. Acid squanders a result of nourishment. These are profoundly acidic, and acidosis is one of the numerous patrons that lead to maturing and the improvement of the disease. The body can discharge acid waste through pee and blood. Whatever isn't emitted will be flowing in the blood. The acid waste amasses and stops up vessels and veins. Along these lines, the cells in the body become oxygen denied and are rendered dormant of multiplication.

- Signs that I have to reestablish my PH
- Low energy, ceaseless weariness
- Nasal blockage

- Visit colds, influenza, and diseases
- Abundance mucous generation
- Neuritis
- Joint torment of joint pain
- Migraines
- Arrangement of pimples, for example, ovarian sores, polycystic ovaries, kindhearted bosom blisters (fibrocystic bosoms)
- Powerless nails, dry hair, dry skin
- Apprehensive, focused, peevish, restless, unsettled
- Muscle torment
- Feel better after a detox diet
- Hives
- Leg issues and fits
- Gastric issues, acid heartburn

Easy to Make Simple Detox Tea Recipes

Before long, it will spring again and time for us to cleanse our bodies and particularly our livers. During this season, it is excellent to give your liver a lift to set it up for the work it should complete. There is one manner by which you can cleanse your liver in availability, and that is by utilizing homegrown teas, in addition to the fact that they are anything but difficult to use the give a fantastic punch to stirring your liver.

One such homegrown definition is designated "Puri-Tea" given by a botanist in Colorado by the name of Brigitte Mars it contains the accompanying fixings:-

- Peppermint, Red Clover, Fennel, Liquorice
- Knives, Dandelion, Oregon Grape Root, Burdock Root
- Butternut Bark, Chickweed, Parsley Root, Nettles
- Or on the other hand, you could attempt this homegrown tea:-
- 1 Part Fennel Seed and 1 Part Fenugreek
- 1 Part Flax Seed and ¼ Par Liquorice Root
- ¼ Part Burdock and 1 Part Peppermint

A further natural blend which is additionally useful for purging and detoxifying the liver is as per the following:

- Yellow Dock Root, Dandelion Root, Liquorice Root
- Red Sage, Sarsaparilla, Hyssop
- Pau de Arco, Milk Thistle Seed, Parsley Leaf

In any case, there are likewise different things that you can do to support your liver also. As a matter of first importance, buy some concentrate of Milk Thistle Seed, and afterward, when you make one of the teas that I have recorded above, include 2-3 full droppers of the focus to it.

Beneath, I likewise give data on what impacts the herbs utilized above in the teas have on the body.

Fennel Seeds help with white cell arrangement in the blood and keep your acid and alkaline levels adjusted. Peppermint is great to use as a body cleanser and toner, while Red Clover is reasonable for blood purging. Licorice is perfect for invigorating the adrenal organs in the body, and Cleavers is an enemy of disease herb. At that point, we have Dandelion, which is useful for purging and fortifying the body. Next comes Oregon Grape Root, which is likewise helpful for purifying and building the body, while Burdock Root is helpful in utilizing refining the body's framework. Concerning Nettles, they are plentiful in minerals that all organizations need. At that point, there is Fenugreek, which disposes of bodily fluid and poisons from the body, while the Yellow Dock Root is excellent not just as a purging specialist for the body however assists with the white cell development. At that point at long last, we have Milk Thistle Seed, which is likewise useful for purging the organization and building its quality.

In any case, on the off chance that you don't wish to make these teas yourself, you can go to any Health Food Store, and they will have them prepared arranged. Yet, a way I would prescribe to set up your very own, it purchases ½ to 1 oz of every herb that you will utilize then in a container place a tablespoon of everyone and shake the substance up and its prepared to use.

At the point when you wish to set up some this tea initially bubble one and ¼ cups of filtered water in a glass compartment, at that point include a piled tablespoon of the blend, enable it to sit for around 10-15 minutes at that point strain and drink once it has cooled adequately. You should drink a cup of this blend before your morning meal and before your feast at night for around 1 to 2 months.

www.ingramcontent.com/pod-product-compliance
Lightning Source LLC
Chambersburg PA
CBHW060834220526
45466CB00003B/1105